# THE NEW ERA OF AIDS

# INTERNATIONAL LIBRARY OF ETHICS, LAW, AND THE NEW MEDICINE

VOLUME 15

*The titles published in this series are listed at the end of this volume.*

# THE NEW ERA OF AIDS

## HIV and Medicine in Times of Transition

*by*

### Christine Kopp

*Department of Social Anthropology,
University of Bern, Switzerland and
Swiss Federal Office of Public Health,
Bern, Switzerland*

## KLUWER ACADEMIC PUBLISHERS
### DORDRECHT / BOSTON / LONDON

A C.I.P. Catalogue record for this book is available from the Library of Congress.

ISBN 1-4020-1048-6

Published by Kluwer Academic Publishers,
P.O. Box 17, 3300 AA Dordrecht, The Netherlands.

Sold and distributed in North, Central and South America
by Kluwer Academic Publishers,
101 Philip Drive, Norwell, MA 02061, U.S.A.

In all other countries, sold and distributed
by Kluwer Academic Publishers,
P.O. Box 322, 3300 AH Dordrecht, The Netherlands.

*Printed on acid-free paper*

For Alex

"Combination therapies probably open up a new era now. That's something that has to be communicated, although it will not gain ground through communication, but through individual examples which are being experienced by people. That's the reality, that's more important than anything we discuss here. We might be moving from the early times – the primeval times, so to speak – to the new era now, but that is something everybody has to be prepared for by himself, prepared to experience it." (Markus Mader)

"For me, I would say, HIV is a difficulty I have to surmount, it's another difficulty in life. I'm lucky enough that I have lived with it for a long time, and I don't think it's gonna kill me in the foreseeable future. Beyond, I think, it will kill me. If I die of something, it will probably be that. – I mean: WHEN I die of something." (Eliane Dutoit)

# CONTENTS

## TABLES

## FIGURES

# ACKNOWLEDGMENTS

This book is based on the invaluable help and support of many people. Fundamental to conducting the research were the people with HIV, the physicians and complementary therapists that kindly agreed to be interviewed and to fill out questionnaires. Although they have to remain anonymous, I would like to express my gratitude for their openness and their patience, for the ideas, insight, fears and hopes they shared with us.

Jan von Overbeck was willing to employ a future anthropologist in a clinic, never questioning the uses of a science as unpractical as anthropology in a setting as efficient as a clinic. His open mind and adventurous spirit opened the path for this book, based on my thesis, and for the project they are developed from. Much of the work within the project was done by my colleague Stefan Lang to whom I am most grateful for several years of collaboration, for new research approaches, and – of course – for insight into the world of computers. Prof. Hans-Ruedi Wicker, the supervisor of my thesis, has been supporting my academic work for many years, starting from research in Paraguay all the way to research in the clinic. I am most grateful for his support and his confidence. I also thank Prof. Wolfgang Marschall for kindly agreeing to become the second examiner of my thesis. Prof. Jean Benoist of the Laboratoire d'Écologie Humaine et d'Anthropologie, Université Aix-Marseille, invited me to his institute, and I am grateful to him and Alice Desclaux for the inspiring discussions of my work during my pleasant stay in Aix-en-Provence. Working at the interface of medicine and anthropology was only possible through people in the clinic who supported our work and collaborated as physicians in different projects: Michèle Schoep always was a dear, calm and competent guide through the world of the clinic. I probably would not have found and followed my way without her. Anne Iten gave me helpful insight into the work of a physician. Hansjakob Furrer's bright thinking clarified many of our ideas and approaches. Prof. Philippe Jaeger, former director of the Outpatient Department of the Inselspital Bern, provided the infrastructure for our projects. The Institut für Ethnologie, Universität Bern, provided the infrastructure to write my thesis, and Christiane Girardin was always helpful with administration and computer support.

Susanne Jost and Alex Sutter read the whole manuscript, and Simone Gretler Heusser, Catherine Moser, Rahel Stuker, Heinzpeter Znoj and Brigit Zuppinger have read parts of it. Denise Choinière once more helped to polish up my English by editing the manuscript. They encouraged me in my work, made valuable comments and suggested improvements for which I thank them very much. With Barbara Krattiger I shared not only the office, but also the ups and downs of her and my work.

Many more provided help in various stages of conducting the research project and writing this book. Amongst them are Marianne Binggeli, Corinne Blöchlinger, Karin Buchs, Susanne Burren, Barbara Federspiel, Josette Guillemin, Ueli Hostettler, Daniel Kessler, Beat Künzi, Kitty Leuzinger, Barbara Lischetti, Monika Lötscher, Christoph Minder, Martin Pavlinec, Marianne Reber, Corina Salis Gross, Silvio Schaller, Jürg Schneider, and Bertino Somaini.

The Swiss National AIDS Research Programme financed the research project this book is based on, and the Research Commission of the Universität Bern supported the writing of the thesis. I thank these institutions for their financial support.

Many dear friends accompanied me during the times when I conducted the balancing act of writing a book as a young mother. Amongst them are: Barbara Orlandini whose dedicated turn towards anthropology encouraged me, Marianne Riedwyl and Irene Leibundgut with whom I did research in the remote fields that characterize anthropology, Lotti Lienhard who has already been a friend for twenty years, Brigit Zuppinger who became so important in such a short time, Beatrice, Kurt, Jonathan, Johanna and Rea Pärli who showed how adventurous family life can be, Andrea Kirchen, Susanne Jost, Tae Woodtli Andrini, Carla Benedetti and Philipp Bleile who all became part of our family life, Bene Totis, Stefan Rieder and Bruno Stadler who have been friends for many years. I am most grateful for the friendship and support of all these people.

My parents, Heidi and Casimir Kopp, never showed any doubts about my strange choice of studies – even if they may have had them. By taking care of Anna, my mother gave me many free hours to work on this book. I thank my parents, my sister Barbara Kaufmann and my brother Christian Kopp for everything they did for me.

Although combining academic work and family life may not always be easy, it is this very combination that I found most inspiring. I thank our beloved children Anna Milena and Basil Xaver for showing me again and again new and wonderful facets of life. Finally, I thank Alex Sutter who helped me in numerous ways. He encouraged me when I felt like giving up, he shares family life and work with me, and he gave some of the most helpful academic input, always with the skeptic mind of the philosopher. This book is dedicated to Alex.

# INTRODUCTION

Ethnographies are almost inevitably introduced[1] by a description of the anthropologist's arrival in the field, "the initial reception by the inhabitants, the slow, agonizing process of learning the language and overcoming rejection, the anguish and loss of leaving" (Pratt 1986: 31). This personal narrative takes a somewhat different turn when the field is a large university hospital in Switzerland, just a short walk from the ethnographer's home[2], and the ethnographer thus cannot rely on the fascination of the exotic when presenting herself to her readers.

I entered the clinic for what eventually turned out to be almost five years of part-time work at the HIV outpatient department in what is probably a paradigmatic way for an anthropologist, that is, by coincidence and connections. I was initially employed as a counselor for the Anonymous HIV Counseling and Testing Center where my work gave me a faint idea of what it must feel like to be a physician. This included the power and responsibility that resulted from the astonishing openness and confidence which persons coming to take an HIV test brought to me, my clearly defined role, and my duty to tell them what is right and wrong when trying to protect themselves against an HIV infection. As an ethnographer, I was used to asking questions for the sake of my research interests, or in order to fulfill academic requirements. Here, I was asking questions (knowing the desired answers) for the sake of public health. I subsequently went back to the job of research by transferring to two research projects in the field of HIV which had been designed by physicians. Assessing and evaluating the research data again confronted me with the different cultures of anthropology and medicine, this time at the level of scientific methods. As can be expected of an anthropologist, I gradually immersed myself in the new culture. The "slow, agonizing process of learning the language" (though luckily not having to overcome rejection) that Pratt described culminated in my case in the decision to learn a bit of biostatistics as part of the language of medical research. An

---

[1] The present introduction is a revised and extended version of an article entitled "Neither here nor there: the anthropologist back from the clinic" (Kopp 2000).

[2] As Gupta and Ferguson pointed out, a main feature of the classical "field" of research is its spatial separation and its distinction from home: "The very distinction between 'field' and 'home' leads directly to what we call a *hierarchy of purity* of field sites. After all, if the field is most appropriately a place that is 'not home', then some places will necessarily be *more* 'not home' than others" (1997: 13, emphases in original). When adopting such a 'hierarchy of purity', then my field has to be characterized as highly impure – which in turn contradicts the very idea of a hospital.

intensive ten-day course that could be described as a rite of passage revealed some of the basics of a new world of thinking, of expressing meaning and claiming authority and truth. Entering the world of medicine also meant participating to a limited degree in the reciprocity of giving and receiving co-authorship for favors done or alliances established or desired. The furthest this game carried me away from my own field of knowledge was when I became the third author of an abstract called: "CD95 (Fas)-Expression on CD4- and CD8-Lymphocytes of Progressors and Non-Progressors to AIDS" (Harr et al. 1997)[3].

Partially entering a new community and acquiring a new language meant that a whole genre of scientific literature suddenly made more sense to me, or at times revealed its nonsense, and gave me the keys to presenting our work to a medical audience according to its standards. At the same time it became more difficult to find a common language with anthropologists. As a researcher, I therefore found myself in a somewhat liminal situation as described by Turner: "neither here nor there; he is betwixt and between the positions assigned by law, custom, convention and ceremonial" (1969: 95). Singer brilliantly describes the ambiguity of clinical anthropology in a chapter asking: "How Critical Can Clinical Anthropology Be?" (1995: 351-370). Facing a rather lonesome position as a social scientist, the anthropologist is driven by the desire to gain legitimacy in the eyes of her colleagues, the medical practitioners, she engages in medical discourse, and her attempts to study the medical arena might turn out to be more difficult than studying the less powerful patients. In a diary entry dating January 29, 1998, I wondered about my role as an anthropologist in a field as political and controversial as HIV/AIDS[4]. The list included: The anthropologist as a foreign body in the clinic – The anthropologist as the advocate of the patient – The anthropologist as a mediator – The anthropologist who herself needs a good physician – The anthropologist who wishes her work was as clear and needed as the physician's. The list of the anthropologist may be extended.

Just when anthropology started to become more exotic than the familiar clinical setting, a turn back toward anthropology was taken through a proposal to the National AIDS Research Programme that was based upon anthropological premises. The project was designed and carried out by fellow anthropologist, Stefan Lang, and myself in collaboration with the physicians Anne Iten, Hansjakob Furrer, and Jan von Overbeck, and headed by Prof. Hans-Rudolf Wicker from the Institut für Ethnologie of the Universität Bern. Formally, it was thus affiliated with the Institut für Ethnologie while we continued to work at the Inselspital in Bern, again symbolizing the fruitful and ambiguous balancing act between anthropology and medicine.

---

[3] (No, I cannot explain what CD95 (fas)-expression is all about.)

[4] HIV stands for Human Immunodeficiency Virus, AIDS for Acquired Immune Deficiency Syndrome.

The project aimed at exploring health care and treatment of people with HIV mainly outside the specialized HIV departments in hospitals and clinics. While at least quantitative data is routinely assessed in the clinical setting, very little is known about the situation amongst general practitioners and complementary therapists, an imbalance that our project attempted to correct. Based upon our evaluation, we provided starting points for improving health care around HIV (Kopp and Lang 1999; Kopp et al. 1998a; 1998b). While our research also included complementary therapists, I will in the following concentrate on our work amongst persons with HIV and general practitioners.

Either through luck or intuition (but I assume it was the former), our research was carried out during the time of the most dramatic changes persons with HIV, doctors and researchers in HIV had faced to date, i.e. during the period in between the 11th International Conference on AIDS 1996 in Vancouver and the 12th World AIDS Conference 1998 in Geneva. In industrialized countries such as Switzerland (Egger et al. 1997), a new generation of antiretroviral drugs, the protease inhibitors, in combination with the already known antiretroviral medication, were for the first time capable of favorably influencing the course of the infection on a broad level. In short, dramatically fewer people in Europe and Northern America were becoming sick with AIDS and dying. The reports of people who had resigned themselves to the reality of an early death and now were challenged by the need to develop new life perspectives became popular (Johnson 1997). Meanwhile, people with HIV also feared being redefined from activists to patients (Hirsch 1997). The 1996 11th International Conference on AIDS[5], the first one I personally attended, was characterized by euphoria over the new treatment possibilities. HIV specialists carried the euphoria home to their clinics whence it subsequently trickled down to per-

---

[5] International AIDS conferences, taking place annually from 1985 to 1994 and then changed to a biannual rhythm, are a powerful and highly sponsored social enactment of current tendencies and debates in HIV/AIDS research. As Feldman noted, based on fieldwork amongst AIDS doctors: "The experience of communitas is not lost forever to my informants but is now integrated into an annual ritual known as the International AIDS Conference" (1995: 183). Besides researchers, also people with HIV populate these conferences as a compulsory, although preferably marginal component which does not always suit the scientists. Treichler cited Robert Gallo complaining about "the amount of diversity" at the 1989 conference in Montreal: "You can't even find the people you want to talk to anymore" (1992: 78). It is probably the social and ritual quality of the conferences that makes them attractive also for fieldwork by social scientists such as Feldman and Treichler. In reviewing science and technology studies, Hess found ethnographic research to increasingly move from the laboratory into a variety of new settings, including conferences. He interpreted this move as reflecting the shift from studying the social construction of scientific facts toward the cultural reconstruction of scientific discourses as they diffuse through scientific and nonscientific communities. In studying the latter, Hess found conferences "a crucial site for ethnographic research. Unlike the laboratory, the conference provides a setting in which the research community is assembled, social and ideological divisions are often clearly evident, and affected publics may also have their voices." (1992: 15). The description similarly reflects my own impression of AIDS conferences.

sons with HIV and into general practices, to be received, revised, rejected, and resisted. By the 1998 12th World AIDS Conference in Geneva, researchers had been sobered of hopes that the new drugs might cure the infection, and a more pessimistic discourse around drug resistance, treatment failure, and the inaccessibility of the new drugs to most people with HIV living outside of Europe and Northern America was predominant. Possibly this more pessimistic discourse was anticipated and accentuated by our interview partners and the people responding to our questionnaire who to some degree looked at the developments from the margins. Most of the physicians worked outside the specialized HIV centers, and people with HIV not only looked back over a prolonged experience with their infection, but their favorable course of infection also allowed them a critical distance toward medical treatment[6].

The research thus captures a crucial moment of transition in HIV/AIDS brought about by the introduction of new treatment options. As the image of HIV was changed from a lethal to a potentially chronic disease, people with HIV and their physicians, both representing the users' side of scientific knowledge, were trying to make sense of the sickness and struggled to position themselves in the face of the ongoing changes.

While I develop my work from a central moment in the history of HIV/AIDS, I do so not only through the eyes of mainly rather critical study populations, but also from a geographically marginal perspective. Switzerland is not precisely a global center of HIV/AIDS research. While at least in biomedical research it gained considerable reputation through the Swiss HIV Cohort Study SHCS (Francioli 1999; Ledergerber et al. 1994), little anthropological research in this field is generated here. There are some disadvantages to this fact, most notably a relative isolation as a researcher. Yet the perspective from the margins may to some degree also support the researcher in keeping, like her interview partners, a critical distance towards the changing trends – both in biomedical and in anthropological research.[7]

The study combines, as outlined in chapter 1, qualitative with quantitative data[8], narration with numbers, providing a configuration that is rather unusual for anthropological research. The methods applied were partly chosen with regard to content,

---

[6] For a detailed description of our study populations, see chapter 1.2.

[7] For further reflections on the role of the "field" in contemporary research and on the relationship between the global anthropological center and its periphery, see chapter 7.

[8] For a discussion of such a combination, see Bryman (1988). One of the rare anthropological examples involving such a combination is Lock's research on the menopause in Japan and the United States (Lock 1993b).

and partly, even though this aspect is usually not mentioned, to strategy[9]. On the strategic level, we wanted to combine the language of anthropology with the language of medical research. More important were the reasons with regard to content: The conditions that limit or favor HIV transmission, the representation of the sickness as well as its treatment and care are not subject to disciplinary boundaries (Benoist and Desclaux 1996). We thus tried to overcome these boundaries by collaborating with physicians, working within the medical setting, and by combining methods from both fields.

On a theoretical level, we quite crudely took as our point of departure the "explanatory model" approach developed by Kleinman (1980) in his milestone book on medical anthropology, an approach that has been used over and over in applied research in the field of medicine. It may hardly be surprising that this point of departure soon proved to be too narrow[10]. Theories of the body and its role in constructing self and sickness as well as research into science and biomedicine as a social and cultural system[11], broadened my view of our research topic. Most importantly, they helped me understand the intense negotiations over boundaries, power, competence, and control addressed by our interview partners.

While many themes as well as part of the underlying concepts changed during the course of this research in accordance to what our interview partners told us, we stuck to the belief that studying HIV and health care from an anthropological perspective cannot be limited to the patient and her perspective of illness, giving her the status of the subjective, the irrational, the non-compliant, the unpredictable factor that distorts medical objectivity and health care, thus implicitly assuming that medicine would be so easy if physicians just did not have to deal with patients. Instead, we treated people with HIV and physicians equally, interviewing both and asking the same type of questions. Not surprisingly in the light of an increasing body of research on biomedicine, we found that the "problem patient" might be the physician himself[12], and his non-compliance may be just as rational as the one of his patients.

Instead of focusing on the doctor-patient interaction, we interviewed people with HIV and their physicians separately. The reasons for this choice were manifold:

---

[9] According to Rouse, networks of scientific communication "shape both what needs to be said and what vocabulary and technical resources can be appropriately utilized" (1992: 11).

[10] As Kleinman himself commented: "Clinically the explanatory model approach may continue to be useful, but ethnography has fortunately moved well beyond this early formulation" (1995: 9).

[11] Part of this research cumulated in the "science wars" fought between researchers from the social sciences and scientists over the authority in science (Fujimura 1998).

[12] Physicians are still mainly male: 88% of our random sample of 542 general practitioners were men.

firstly, not all persons with HIV are patients, and we wanted to include non-patients as well. Secondly, sick people spend only a small fraction of their time in the role of the patient, and studying the doctor-patient interaction only captures a narrow aspect of the experience of being sick (Conrad 1987). This observation may be especially true in the case of people with a long-term asymptomatic sickness such as HIV. Thirdly, a decreasing fraction of the work of the doctor is determined by his interaction with the patient. Instead, there are specialist consultations, laboratory results, or economic and political negotiations which gain in importance. As a consequence, medicine moves increasingly away from the patient. It might therefore provide more insight into health care to analyze, say, the interactions between physicians and representatives of pharmaceutical companies visiting them in their practices than to observe the doctor-patient interaction.

Our methodological decision was strengthened by the observation that the introduction of the new combination therapies rapidly increased the importance of basic science, specialized medicine, treatment guidelines and laboratory tests. As we conducted our study, the image of HIV/AIDS as a lethal condition had been transformed into "the view of 96/97, that means, a chronic sickness with the need to take medication, but without deterioration", as the physician Claude Keller expressed it. These rapid changes in the field of HIV reflect and accentuate broader changes in medicine and health care, some of which I tried to trace in my work. In the following paragraphs, I only roughly sketch the different aspects of these processes which are elaborated in chapters 2 to 6 of this book.

For the person infected with HIV, the development of a new identity circles around re-establishing personal integrity, autonomy, and control in the face of the potentially uncontrollable virus, the "ghost" as David Burki put it, within the body. The immune system receives symbolic value as the body's network for distinguishing between self and other and for organizing rejection, integration, and adaptation. It thus becomes the physical expression of the struggle for integrity and control. In chapter 2, I outline these processes and relate them to virological and immunological constructions of HIV/AIDS and its interaction with the infected body.

The struggle over autonomy and control is also carried over into the health care process, where it became highly accentuated with the therapeutic power of the physician through antiretroviral combination therapies. As I argue in chapter 3 where I look at the changing doctor-patient relation, treatment brought power back to medicine, but this power does not necessarily translate into new asymmetry in the doctor-patient interaction and new authority for the physician. Rather, there are specialist consultations, laboratory results, or economic and political negotiations which gain importance.

In chapter 4, I focus on the usage of antiretroviral treatment in the general practice and by people with HIV as it shifts from experimental to standard therapy. Our data indicate that patients and general practitioners seemed to be more reluctant to use and prescribe antiretroviral treatment than recommended by scientists and guidelines and practiced by physicians at specialized HIV centers. Based on our research, I try to elucidate physicians' and patients' motives against prescribing or using treatment.

In chapter 5, I explore the struggles between generalists and specialists over their respective fields of competence. I argue that the redefinition of the general practitioner's and the specialist's role in health care, as negotiated and articulated in the field of HIV/AIDS, might ultimately lead to a division of the patient, with the patient as "person" assigned to the general practitioner and the patient as "body" to the specialist.

With the new power of antiretroviral therapies, basic and clinical science gain importance in HIV care and are expected to guide the work of the individual physician. In chapter 6, I describe how large-scale initiatives in medicine aiming at an increased integration of the results of clinical science into the daily work of the general practitioner, represented by the approach called "Evidence-Based Medicine" (Sackett et al. 1997), cause fear and resistance amongst a portion of physicians.

As the construction of HIV and the medical care of HIV patients were in transition during our study, this book illuminates some of the central aspects of this transition and shows how they also transcend the field of HIV/AIDS. These aspects include the changing images of sickness and the body, the shifts in the doctor-patient interaction and in the interaction between physicians from different specialties and with different institutional backgrounds, the translation of basic and clinical science into the daily work of the physician, and the increasing demand to base the work of the physician on scientific evidence. HIV/AIDS might be paradigmatic for these processes. As a sickness arousing broad public interest, it is highly symbolically charged, and since it is still a new sickness, it provides an arena where new approaches are developed and adapted by people affected, by public health, science, and medicine.

# CHAPTER 1

# METHODS AND STUDY POPULATIONS

"People with HIV/AIDS are a vulnerable group that should be protected
from researchers."[13]

## 1.1. METHODS: NARRATIVES AND NUMBERS

Anthropologists doing research in the field of medicine are still rather surprising for their research subjects. While psychologists have a clearly defined role within medicine, anthropologists remain, at least in Switzerland, undeterminable, even more so for the physicians than for the patients, as I may illustrate by a passage from my interview with the general practitioner Jonas Ender:

> "On the one hand there are components like in any malignant progressive disease, but where you somehow never really know what is actually going on. (... ). I have this patient with a Polycythaemia vera who... – are you a physician or a psychologist?
>
> ck: Neither nor. An anthropologist, social scientist.
>
> An anthropologist? – Well, I'll have to stop speaking in technical terminology then. Okay, that is somehow a semi-malignant blood disease which can also develop over ten, fifteen years. Well, the blood produces too many red blood corpuscles."

At times, being an anthropologist in medicine became tiresome since it required continuous justifications and explications. Yet the indeterminable status of our profession also bore the advantage that we seemed to be open enough to our interview partners to allow different meanings, attitudes, and explanations to be elaborated on with us. Thus, while we were not clearly positioned in terms of professional background, our connection to the HIV center at the outpatient clinic of a large university hospital did position us in terms of institutional affiliation. On a national level, the HIV centers represent the sources of biomedical knowledge from where it flows to the peripheries of smaller hospitals, general practitioners, patients, and the public.

---

[13] Quoted from Ambrose Rachier, 12th World AIDS Conference, "Bridging Session: Ethics and Science", July 1, 1998.

1

HIV centers therefore occupy a position of power which is both acknowledged and resisted.

Most of my knowledge of the biomedical aspects of HIV/AIDS and its treatment is based on my working within the HIV center, attending rounds, conferences and further education, reading journals and articles passed amongst the team members, and discussing new developments. Based on this fieldwork, I analyze in some chapters of this book how knowledge is produced, established and diffused in medicine through scientific articles and social events, mainly conferences.

Working in an HIV center also influenced my implicit understanding of medical work and of HIV care and treatment. Institutionally, I was closer to the initial enthusiasm about the new combination therapies and the so-called "aggressive" approaches to treatment than the doubts and reluctance I encountered when interviewing general practitioners and people with HIV. When I focus in this book on HIV care provided by general practitioners, I am thus doing so by peering over the boundary between specialized and general medicine. It might be because of the very fact that I kept going back and forth between specialized and general medicine that I increasingly became aware of their struggles over where the boundary is to be drawn and how much autonomy and competence is attributed to each side.

The main two phases of our empirical study involved first interviews and second a questionnaire survey. Further fieldwork though took place after this fieldwork, i.e. when I had moved to the anthropology department to "write up" this text in the classical, though in my case minimal spatial separation from the field (Clifford 1997). Following the themes that emerged in the empirical study into various directions involved data gathering using methods quite different from those that initially characterized the research. Instead of merely writing up, I followed discussions in Internet newsgroups, analyzed media coverage, drug advertisements, or discourses in medical journals. As I remained almost "naturally" connected to these sources, it seemed to make little sense to limit my analysis to the data gathered in the initial research process.

In the first phase of the empirical study, we conducted semi-structured interviews (Britten 1995b; Kiefl 1991) with people with HIV from the Long-Term Survivor Cohort recruited for a former interdisciplinary study on long-term survival (Kopp et al. 1999) and with their health care providers[14]. Physicians tend to be surprised, if not doubtful, when a study is based on interviews and thus attributes ana-

---

[14] Health care providers, as mentioned in the introduction, included orthodox physicians and complementary therapists. As I focus here on orthodox medicine, I will not describe our empirical work with complementary therapists.

lytical status to narratives. Nevertheless, in contradiction to the language of medical science dominated by populations and numbers, the language of medical practice is also based on individuals and narratives, as represented by the medical anamnesis and the medical history (Good 1994; Mattingly 1998)[15]. The narrative though not only holds a weak position in medical research, but also a somewhat ambiguous position in medical practice. With increasing possibilities to look into the body and to extract data from it, i.e. through visual methods or laboratory tests, the narrative receives the status of an unreliable subjective account of what is really going on in the body, an account to be verified, modified or rejected through the objective data provided by biotechnology. Despite this unreliability, the narrative provides a main starting point for the clinical investigation (Hydén 1997), and, after all, an evaluation whether diagnosis and treatment are considered to be effective.

The questions we put together for the interviews covered definition, etiology and course of HIV/AIDS, sources of information on HIV/AIDS, living with HIV or working as a physician with HIV patients, health care, doctor-patient interaction, antiretroviral treatment and compliance/adherence. We discussed the interview questions with anthropologists, a senior physician at an HIV center, a complementary therapist, a general practitioner and an epidemiologist, and subsequently revised the questions based on their feedback.

We conducted at total of eleven interviews with people with HIV and eleven interviews with their physicians. Of these 22 interviews, 13 were conducted by myself and the remaining nine by my colleague Stefan Lang. 18 interviews were held in Swiss German, three in French, and one in English. My colleague and I each tried to interview the same persons with HIV we had already interviewed in the prior project and therefore already knew personally. Each of us subsequently interviewed the physicians caring for the persons with HIV we had interviewed.

The names of our interview partners are pseudonyms. While the mix of names of Swiss German, French, and other European origins should indicate the variety of the people we talked to, they do not represent the origins of the individual interview partners. To further grant our interview partners anonymity, I changed some of the personal attributes of the interview partners.

The interviews lasted between 30 to 90 minutes and were tape-recorded. Interview partners who wished so received a tape and/or a transcript. The interviews initially were transcribed fully and verbatim in their original language, although the

---

[15] The case history as a classic form of presenting medical knowledge provides a middle level between the work with the individual patient and medical science. It represents the standardized way in which individual patient cases are recounted, reflected upon, and generalized.

Swiss German interviews were transcribed in German. All interviews were then thematically indexed and evaluated both by my colleague and myself. For quotation in the text, the language in the shorter interview passages as well as in the narratives introducing each part was polished in an attempt to make it more coherent, thus more resembling a written text. I was strongly asked to do so by interview partners reading the verbatim transcription of their interviews and finding that their spoken language sounded too incoherent when written down word by word. In a final step, the cited passages were translated into English[16].

In the interview passages cited in my text, omissions are indicated with (...) and additions to enhance comprehensibility stand in {brackets}. Since the integration of short, thematically selected interview passages into my own text obscures the internal consistency of the narrative, I chose to recount a selection of narratives more fully. These five narratives from people with HIV and physicians introduce chapters 2 to 6 of this book. Although largely trying to leave the chronological order of the interview, I sometimes changed it in order to increase thematic coherence. Minor additions to enhance comprehensibility are not indicated. The major change I made in these narratives is the construction of a monologue by putting together interview sequences while leaving out the questions of the interviewer. Although I acknowledge authorship for these narratives, I hope with Clifford: "If accorded an autonomous textual space, transcribed at sufficient length, indigenous statements make sense in terms different from those of the arranging ethnographer" (Clifford 1988: 51). It is my aim to accord analytical status to our interview partners (DiGiacomo 1992) instead of reading their narratives as unconscious accounts of social and cultural "rules" beyond their reach and recognition.

I understand the narratives created in the interviews not as an image of events, but a an ongoing retrospective (re-)construction of experience (Skultans 2000), or, as Andrea Meier put it:

> "Now it looks like a trajectory, and back then it was simply behavior, things you did just like that, without reason, no aims or anything. And now I see... now it turns into a trajectory."

Good gave a somewhat similar description of narrative and the relationship between narrative and experience as Andrea Meier: "Narrative is a form in which experience is represented and recounted, in which events are presented as having meaningful and coherent order, in which activities and events are described along with the experiences associated with them and the significance that lends them their sense for the persons involved. But experience always far exceeds its description or narrativization" (1994: 139). He also pointed out that narrators are typically in the

---

[16] Also, passages cited from literature in German are translated into English by the author.

middle of a story which is changing as the events unfold. Both narrative and its interpretation therefore must remain provisional in nature.

Amongst the factors that are involved in the production of a specific narrative are the place where it is recounted, the time when it is recounted, and the particular person(s) it is recounted to and with. Given the different contexts in which a particular person recounts his/her narrative, there are different narratives produced. *The narrative* thus does not exist (Hydén 1997). Good conceptualizes the role of the person participating in the narrative, in our case us as interviewers, through the duality of plot and emplotment. He described "plot as the underlying structure of a story, and 'emplotment' as the activity of a reader of hearer of a story who engages imaginatively in making sense of the theory" (1994: 144). The descriptions and interpretations presented here therefore are my emplotment of the narratives. The interviewers, my colleague and myself, influenced this emplotment as co-authors of the narrative (Williams 1984). In addition, the plot created by the interview partners and the interview setting itself also influenced my emplotment.

We held the interviews with people with HIV at their homes[17] in order to separate the interview from the world of biomedicine and medical institutions. Physicians though were interviewed at their practice[18]. This decision partly corresponds to the role of the physicians as professional caregivers of the people with HIV. Partly it was a practical decision since physicians seem to spend a considerable part of their lives in their practice. The argument may also hide the fact that in the role of an anthropologist-researcher it is more difficult to enter the private sphere of physicians than of people with HIV.

The importance of the temporal dimension, the moment in which the narrative is constructed, is accentuated in our research for two reasons. Firstly, all people with HIV we talked to had been infected before 1991 and looked back over a prolonged experience with HIV. Choosing persons with a prolonged sickness experience is a common approach in research on enduring or chronic conditions (Carricaburu and Pierret 1995; Pierret 1997; Williams 1984) since it provides the opportunity to talk to "seasoned professionals" (Williams 1984: 176). Secondly, as the interviews took place between April and August 1997, shortly after the broad introduction of antiretroviral combination therapies, the narratives were shaped by the contemporary situation which in turn was rapidly changing.

---

[17] With the exception of the interviews with David Burki and Peter Carreira who preferred to come to our office.

[18] An exception was Markus Mader who also chose to come to our office.

In a second phase of our research, we elaborated two questionnaires based on the interview evaluation, one for people with HIV, and the other for general practitioners. Again, we asked people with HIV and their physicians in some cases the same questions, in other cases the same type of question was adapted to their specific situation. The four-page questionnaires covered views of HIV and antiretroviral therapies, doctor-patient interaction, sources of information on HIV, health care and usage of antiretroviral therapies. While we already had detailed socio-demographic data from people with HIV through the Long-Term Survivor Study, the questionnaire for general practitioners also asked for socio-demographic data. Data from the Long-Term Survivor Study on the usage of health care also allowed a prospective comparison between 1995/96 and 1998, thus comparing the situation before and after the wide introduction of antiretroviral combination therapies. The themes, questions and categories used in the questionnaire were derived from the interviews, and the results mainly aimed at providing "a sense of typicality and generality" (Bryman 1988: 143) of a few insights from the interviews.

The questionnaires were discussed with anthropologists, general practitioners, complementary therapists, senior physicians specialized in HIV, epidemiologists and a statistician, and subsequently revised. In a pilot study, the questionnaires were randomly handed out by a secretary to ten HIV patients at the outpatient department of the Inselspital Bern, and mailed to 24 general practitioners. Besides filling out the questionnaires, the pilot study population was asked for a feedback on the questionnaire. We used the pilot study to test the questionnaire for comprehensibility, acceptability, and response rate (16 of 24 general practitioners and six of ten HIV patients). Based on the pilot study, we made a few final adaptations. An external translator translated the German questionnaires into French. The French versions were checked and compared to the German versions by a French native speaker who is a physician specialized in HIV.

Questionnaires were mailed in January/February 1998. General practitioners returned their questionnaires anonymously, and we mailed the questionnaire twice, with different cover letters, to the entire population. Questionnaires to people with HIV were encoded; people not responding received a second questionnaire with a corresponding cover letter, and we subsequently phoned them if they had not returned the second questionnaire.

An external professional provider of data processing entered the questionnaires returned into the computer. We evaluated them in a statistical program for the social sciences (SPSS). Frequency distributions were calculated with the Pearson's Chi Square test. P-values below the 0.05 level of significance were considered as significant.

Slightly earlier than our questionnaire study, another study (Bassetti et al. 1999) assessed prevalence of antiretroviral therapies in HIV centers in a sample of people with HIV from the Swiss HIV Cohort Study SHCS. As they also assessed reasons against prescribing treatment as given by the physicians, we had the possibility to compare some of our data with data from the specialized HIV centers.

As we recruited people with HIV for the Long-Term Survival Study, study participants expressed a demand to receive information on the study and the results (Lang et al. 1996). Besides organizing two meeting days with study participants, we edited over the period of the two studies a total of five *Study News*, bulletins in German and French with information on HIV and our studies, including summaries and translations of scientific articles and the study results. The bulletins were mailed to all study participants as well as to persons and institutions working in the field of HIV/AIDS in Switzerland.

## 1.2. STUDY POPULATIONS

*Interviews*

We interviewed eleven persons with HIV (table 1) and eleven physicians (table 2). People with HIV were chosen from the Long-Terms Survivor Cohort by roughly stratifying them according to sex, mode of transmission, and type of health care. We asked 17 people in order to conduct eleven interviews; six people did not agree to be interviewed either because they were absent during the interview phase (one person), because they psychically felt too unstable (two persons), because they were critical about research in general (one person), and due to reasons not further specified (two persons). It may be assumed that our interview partners were biased for being open to talk about HIV and health care and for feeling stable enough to conduct such an interview. Nevertheless, five of the six persons who did not want to be interviewed filled out the questionnaire in the second phase of the research.

*Table 1. Interview partners – people with HIV*

| Pseudonym | Sex | | Year of birth[19] | Mode of transmission | | | CD4[20] | 1st pos. Test[21] | Health care | | |
|---|---|---|---|---|---|---|---|---|---|---|---|
| | m | f | | IVDU[22] | hetero-sexual | homo sexual | | | HIV center | GP[23] | CT[24] |
| Jeff Dijon | I | | 1955-59 | (I)[25] | (I) | | 355 | 1988 | | I | |
| David Burki | I | | 1960-64 | | | I | 738 | 1986 | I | | |
| Jana Seifert | | I | 1965-69 | | I | | 460 | 1987 | | I | |
| Andrea Meier | | I | 1965-69 | | I | | 481 | 1989 | | I | I |
| Erich Roth | I | | 1950-54 | | | I | 470 | 1985 | | I | I |
| Salvatore Annoni | I | | 1960-64 | | | I | 425 | 1986 | | I | |
| Moritz Pedrini | I | | 1930-34 | | | I | 354 | 1989 | | I | I |
| Peter Carreira | I | | 1940-44 | | | I | 428 | 1985 | | I | |
| Eliane Dutoit | | I | 1955-59 | I | | | 495 | 1988 | I | | |
| Simone Peyer | | I | 1965-69 | | I | | 1251 | 1989 | | | |
| Jakob Theiler[26] | I | | 1950-54 | I | | | 401 | 1988 | I | | |
| Total | 7 | 4 | | 2/(3) | 3/(4) | 5 | | | 3 | 8 | 3 |

The physicians we interviewed were the health care providers of the people with HIV we had interviewed. They were asked for an interview based on a written informed consent by their patients. All of the physicians agreed to be interviewed. Eight of the physicians worked in private practice, one was an assistant physician and two were senior physicians in HIV centers. All but one physician were men, and they also all had experience with HIV/AIDS patients other than our interview partners. In contrast to most physicians working in a private practice who were general practitioners, Claude Keller was specialized in infectious diseases and mainly cared for HIV/AIDS patients. Among the general practitioners interviewed, François Neher, though presently not caring for a high number of HIV/AIDS patients, and

---

[19] In order to further preserve the participants' anonymity, I indicate the time span of five years in which the person was born instead of giving the precise year.

[20] CD4-cells/µl as measured during the Long-Term Survivor Study visit between November 1995 and April 1996.

[21] Year of the first test verified by written reference.

[22] IVDU stands for intravenous drug use.

[23] The abbreviation "GP" used in tables and figures stands for "general practitioner".

[24] Complementary therapist

[25] Mode of transmission is unclear, but (I) indicates the possible modes.

[26] The interview was held together with his wife, who is also HIV-positive, and whom I named Alice Theiler.

Gregor Pfister were according to our knowledge the most experienced in HIV/AIDS care.

*Table 2. Interview partners – physicians*

| Pseudonym | Sex | | Prof. position (since when) | | HIV/AIDS patients last 12 months[27] |
|---|---|---|---|---|---|
| | m | f | HIV center | private practice | |
| Franz Jann | I | | Intern (1995) | | 50 |
| Jonas Ender | I | | | I (1989) | 2 |
| André Favre | I | | | I (1989) | 5 |
| François Neher | I | | | I (1983) | 3-8 |
| Markus Mader | I | | | I (1987) | 4 |
| Luca Granges | I | | SP[28] (?) | | ? |
| Gregor Pfister | I | | | I (1988) | 40 |
| Marco Deville | I | | | I (1981) | 8 |
| Andreas Bauer | I | | SP (1995) | | 30 |
| Claude Keller | I | | | I (1995) | 380 |
| Isabelle Aguet | | I | | I (1997) | 4 |
| Total | 10 | 1 | 3 | 8 | |

*Questionnaires*

The questionnaires were mailed to the following populations:
-   People with HIV (n=50) from the Long-Term Survivor Cohort
Inclusion criteria in 1995 were: first positive test with written reference ≤1990, CD4 ≥500 cells/µl, no antiretroviral medication taken. Of the 56 persons participating in the study in 1995/96, three had died for reasons other than AIDS and three could not be found anymore.
-   General practitioners (n=804)
We sent the questionnaire to a random sample of 1/6 of the population (3 of the 807 questionnaires mailed were undeliverable) of physicians with a FMH title[29] in either

---

[27] The number indicates the estimated number of HIV/AIDS patients over the 12 months prior to the interview.

[28] Senior physician

[29] On its homepage, the FMH describes itself and the FMH title as follows: "The FMH - Foederatio Medicorum Helveticorum/Swiss Medical Association is the umbrella organisation for Swiss physicians. (…). One of the main objectives of the Swiss Medical Association (FMH) is the regulation and supervision of the education of medical interns after they complete state examinations. This further education usually results in the award of the title of FMH medical specialist (or 'Facharzttitel' known previously as 'Spezialartzttitel')" (http://www.fmh.ch/fmh.cfm, June 9, 2000).

General or Internal Medicine and working in a private practice (n=4'840 according to our set of addresses).

*Table 3. Questionnaire response*

| Study group | Mailed (n) | Response (n) | Response (%) |
|---|---|---|---|
| People with HIV | 50 | 46 | 92 |
| General practitioners | 804 | 542 | 67.4 |

The response rate among people with HIV was with 92% very high, which is probably due to the fact that we knew everybody personally through the former study, that we had always informed them about the studies through our *Study News*, and that we personally talked to them when not responding the questionnaire. The response rate of 67.4% among the general practitioners is also satisfactory.

*Table 4. Socio-demographic characteristics of people with HIV (part A)*

|  | n | Valid % |
|---|---|---|
| **Sex** | | |
| Female | 22 | 47.8 |
| Male | 24 | 52.2 |
| **Mode of transmission** | | |
| Intravenous drug use | 15 | 32.6 |
| Homosexual | 15 | 32.6 |
| Heterosexual | 10 | 21.7 |
| Heterosexual or I.V. drug use | 6 | 13.0 |
| **Mother tongue** | | |
| French | 20 | 43.5 |
| German | 18 | 39.1 |
| Italian | 2 | 4.3 |
| Other | 6 | 13.0 |
| **Income[30]** | | |
| Low | 2 | 4.4 |
| Lower middle | 17 | 37.8 |
| Upper middle | 7 | 15.6 |
| Upper | 19 | 42.2 |

*Table 5. Socio-demographic characteristics of people with HIV (part B)*

|  | n | Mean | Median | Std. Deviation | Minimum | Maximum |
|---|---|---|---|---|---|---|
| Year of birth | 46 | 1959 | 1961 | 6.9 | 1932 | 1969 |
| Year of 1st positive HIV test | 46 | 1987 | 1986 | 1.6 | 1983 | 1990 |
| Self-reported CD4 values 1998 (cells/μl) | 37 | 697 | 610 | 321 | 214 | 1'457 |
| Self-reported viremia (copies/ml) | 34 | 22'029 | 98 | 45'374 | 0 | 180'000 |

---

[30] The income was calculated in correspondence with the indicators (as of October 4th, 1994) used by the *Bundesamt für Statistik Abteilung Bevölkerung und Beschäftigung* in the *"Schweizerischen Gesundheitsbefragung 1992/93"*. Income is calculated according to the following model: Income = monthly gross household income divided by equivalent figure of the number of persons living in the household (equivalent figure: 1st adult=1, each additional adult=0.5, each child ≤14 years=0.3). The income categories were built as follows: 1: low income≤1'399 SFr.; 2: lower middle income=1'400 SFr - 2'999 Fr.; 3: upper middle income=3'000 – 3'749 SFr.; 4: upper income≥3'750 SFr..

The study group of people with HIV is well balanced according to sex and mode of transmission. It represents the different language groups in Switzerland and different levels of income. The mean year of birth is 1959 and the mean year of infection 1987. Due to the recruitment criteria (see above), the group is characterized by having a prolonged experience with HIV and a relatively stable course of the infection with favorable laboratory values without taking antiretroviral treatment up to 1995. The study group is thus not to be considered as representative for the population of people with HIV in Switzerland. Yet with antiretroviral combination therapies, an increasing number of people with HIV are now in the position of living with a relatively stable course of their infection and without symptoms for a prolonged period of time. They thus are in a situation which is to some degree comparable to the one of our study group.

*Table 6. Socio-demographic characteristics of general practitioners (part A)*

|  | n | Valid % |
| --- | --- | --- |
| Sex |  |  |
| Male | 475 | 88.3 |
| Female | 63 | 11.7 |
| Medical education |  |  |
| General medicine | 376 | 69.9 |
| Internal medicine | 149 | 27.7 |
| Other | 13 | 2.4 |
| Additional education in complementary therapies |  |  |
| Yes | 56 | 10.3 |
| No | 486 | 89.7 |
| Language of questionnaire[31] |  |  |
| French | 126 | 23.2 |
| German | 416 | 76.8 |

---

[31] The database did not contain information on mother tongue. We chose to send questionnaires in the language corresponding to the geographical area. To general practitioners living in areas where both French and German is spoken as well as to general practitioners living in the Italian part of Switzerland, we sent both the French and the German version and left it to the general practitioners' choice which questionnaire they wanted to fill out and return. The language was classified according to the language of the questionnaires returned.

*Table 7. Socio-demographic characteristics of general practitioners (part B)*

|  | n | Mean | Median | Std. Deviation | Minimum | Maximum |
|---|---|---|---|---|---|---|
| Year of birth | 538 | 1949 | 1950 | 8.3 | 1918 | 1964 |
| Year of opening private practice | 531 | 1984 | 1985 | 8.3 | 1951 | 1997 |

The high percentage of men among the general practitioners represented the situation in the total population of physicians specialized in General or Internal Medicine and working in a private practice in Switzerland: As of 1998, 90% of these physicians specialized in General Medicine and 88% specialized in Internal Medicine were men. Similarly, the mean age of 49 years (year of birth 1949) in our population corresponded exactly to the mean age of physicians working in a private practice in 1998. In contrast, given that the total number of physicians specialized in Internal Medicine and working in a private practice (2'895) is higher than the number of physicians specialized in General Medicine and working in a private practice (2'505), the latter are with 69.9% overrepresented in our sample (Generalsekretariat der Verbindung der Schweizer Ärztinnen und Ärzte FMH 1999). 10.3% of the general practitioners in our population have an additional education in complementary therapy, most frequently in homeopathy (n=14) and acupuncture (n=12), the remaining being distributed over a great variety of approaches. A majority (76.8%) of the general practitioners in our population live in the German-speaking part of Switzerland. The mean year of opening a private practice is 1984.

# CHAPTER 2

# BODIES AND BOUNDARIES

## MORITZ PEDRINI: THE IMMUNITY REDUCTION OF OPPRESSED PEOPLE[32]

In the beginning, in the whole first phase of coping almost with a shock, I was with Doctor X who had just opened his practice. And that was always very nice. He was very sensitive and so he became our family doctor. Then, when I realized that I am actually not doing badly and when I saw that I should do something to do even better, I chose to do everything I heard of. First it was homeopathy with an iridologist, that means he makes his diagnosis by looking at the iris. He right away gave me a lot of homeopathic globule and they helped me remarkably. I developed a very good feeling for my body, and I could – as I remember – bike again with pleasure and so on. And then I heard that the anthroposophists could enhance immunity in cancer mainly with *Iscador*, a mistletoe drug, also a homeopathic thing. I think it is mainly a drug against cancer which can also partly be explained through immunity reduction. So I went and was passed on to a Doctor Y who right away said: yes, we do have some experience with it. And ever since – that was maybe eight, no, seven years ago – I always regularly injected it twice a week, with short breaks, once I paused for a month and a half. That was mistletoe, and a few other things. (...). And then some time ago, maybe two years ago, I realized that the *Roche*-drug *Berocca* is very good for me. Not taking very much of it, not regularly at all, let's say twice or three times a week half a tablet, that's really not much. And then I realized that half an Aspirin helped when I for example didn't sleep well. And very often I felt I had to take a vitamin combination. I suspect that this vitamin combination has always had such a clear effect on me, already for 20 or 25 years, especially on days when I have to assert myself in my work, it makes me capable in a good way and I am absolutely in best shape, I believe it could be because it contains iodide. That's my lay opinion, because this iodide is not found in most other drugs. (...). Further approaches were following more the psychological side. First of all, I realized that it is very important to me to work along the lines pursued by my two rather long-lasting psychotherapies, analytical therapies. And now, a bit more than a year ago, in spring a year ago, I went to an analyst I already knew and already had a good understanding with, and I started therapy with him, about once a week or every two weeks, and that lasted for almost a year. But the essential problem treated there

---

[32] The narrative is – in contrast to the narratives introducing the following parts – barely revised by myself. Following an introductory question, Moritz Pedrini told his story as I reproduce it here (only omitting a few short passages), without being asked any further questions. He seemed to have the whole story already waiting in his mind. After the long narrative passage, the interview went on with further questions and answers.

was the problem of my relation with the school, my situation there and the whole background to this relation going back to my youth, my childhood. Somehow to look again how it developed, where I could try to omit the same reactions, where I could begin something new and much more differentiated. And that was very important since I realized that I longed to liberate myself from the school because my entry into the school did not happen under optimal circumstances. First of all, as a child I was not necessarily talented in painting, I had a strong idea of art and a desire, but the talent was not so clear. It was rather due to the circumstances that I eventually decided for art. And now it turned out that ever since my childhood there was a certain pressure that I should paint. Like many children who first under a certain pressure... – seen from the exterior, the pressure was not all that big, but there were always challenges and decisions: either you paint, or we stop the lessons. And in that way, the whole thing was a bit uneasy. That was the world of my mother anyway and I did not feel very comfortable about it. Well, the whole thing pointed towards a profession that I might not have chosen under very normal circumstances. I might have turned into a very interested amateur, I might have become an artist anyhow, that's not so clear, but in that case it would have been under different conditions, with more freedom, at least as I hope. But maybe that's all an illusion, too. But in any case I believe that remnants of this pressure have always been carried on from one situation to the other, without my ability to become fully aware of them or removing them. And so I understood now that I am very relieved because I can start to retire already. And what is interesting, the first consequence of my relief was that when I came to see you[33], to take blood tests, that they turned out quite worse than the ones just half a year before which were above 600, and then suddenly 360 or something, the helper cells I mean. And I actually felt well. It was only during the summer right after that, last summer, that so many duties had piled up again that I actually felt almost worse than ever before. I felt very old, felt I was trembling inside, and, sometimes, just very exhausted. But that summer the helper cells had climbed again above 400, around 450, and ever since one problem after the other gradually got resolved. First of all I had the exhibit, and I also held a speech that was appreciated. And now I have another exhibit that will cost me a lot of work, and I feel very well that it will mean the end of everything I *must* do. I will be able to freely decide absolutely every moment whether I work or not. (...). And for that reason my relationship with the school never was ideal, for the pressure hindered my artistic development and therefore I didn't get the response I imagined I should get to correspond to my artistic and pedagogical ideals. And now, with the retirement I now await calmly, and with the psychotherapy I recently finished, I feel that I will start a new phase in life in which for the first time there is nothing I have to do. And this often mainly means that I have the time to sleep when I am tired. (...). What I find very important is biking, going for a walk. I regularly need certain physical training tasks, and then I am – I have the feeling that I am also safe in relation to the infection. (...). I have, to resume the whole thing, I also have a comprehensive idea which in part is also critical of society. I think with some reservation it can generally be accepted. Through my sexual orientation I have the disposition to be opposed to the official, the conventional lifestyle. But also besides that I believe that I have enough reason to criticize the paternalistic orientation of our society. And that is something which seems very important to me. Now I have a purpose in the political, the artistic, and also in the pedagogical and the practical domain, since I will also keep on teaching, just not regularly anymore. The purpose to introduce everywhere the *weltanschauung* that you should not orient so much towards measurable values, that you should not demand results from people, but instead that the results are allowed to come by themselves

---

[33] He refers to his visit for our previous study on non-progression.

since they come much more easily that way. If you want to put it that way, to support people as people in a way that they themselves learn to enjoy the essence of art instead of first having to learn the artistic techniques as an end in themselves. These are things that have actually long been condemned but in practice they are still decisive. And that you do the same thing in politics, that's also an aim. And the conclusion for HIV – for the whole thing, for this situation as a social syndrome, you could almost say – that I come to is that HIV is actually a socially conditioned sickness, supported through the immunity reduction of oppressed people in an achievement-oriented world, and that's how it could spread. I think that in principle a person who can omit pressure, who can structure his life in a way that he doesn't feel alienated pressure anywhere, that he has a natural capacity to control the virus by himself. It is very interesting that while presently my duties at school come to an end I often forget to either inject *Iscador* or to take my vitamins. And it is very interesting that for the first time in many years I have the feeling that I do not need the experience of homo-erotic sexuality. I suddenly have the feeling that I am a person who can work as an artist, who can think and do things also without a sexual experience. Until last year, until maybe a few months ago, I did not have this feeling, and I directly relate that to the hierarchic situation at school, to the contractual relationship and the very latent, but for a psychologically trained person who is fully aware of his unconscious, absolutely perceptible pressure from above.

* * *

Health has become a central element of personal identity[34] in modernity, and AIDS serves as the paradigmatic sickness to draw the line between the healthy and the polluted (Crawford 1994). A person who is sick has crossed a line that separates her from the healthy others. Identity-building along the lines of health may involve considerable efforts and difficulties already for the healthy ones, as Crawford (1985) vividly described for Americans. The question though receives a new urgency when one is becoming sick, and even more so when the sickness is as stigmatized as HIV/AIDS. While on the level of society, efforts are made to distance ourselves from sickness[35], the individual who is infected with HIV faces the question of how the self can be reconstructed with the virus already within the body, the boundaries of the body already violated. For people with HIV, the experience of infection centers around re-organizing the interface between self and society[36], and organizing the cohabitation with and control of the virus within the body.

---

[34] I agree with Bommes and Scherr in their (rather complicated) definition of identity: "'Identity' in our understanding stands for the need to claim both the continuity of the individual life history and the ability to meaningfully integrate the current individual life practice in the face of biographically and currently heterogeneous circumstances of life and demands on behavior. In that sense, identity is not a natural attribute of individuals, but stands for the attempt to behave towards oneself and the social circumstances of life in a way which allows perceiving the individual biography as continuous and the current life practice as coherent" (1991: 295).

[35] See Kopp (2002) for a review of how boundaries have been and currently are drawn between the healthy and the potentially sick.

[36] As Ariss and Dowsett noted: "Having HIV does not necessarily generate, in itself, a damaged sense of the self. Self is monitored in the context of social relationships" (1997: 56).

From the viewpoint of society, the sick person is first of all a danger to its members. This danger is accentuated when – as in the case of HIV/AIDS – contagion, sexuality, and social deviance such as homosexuality and injecting drug use are combined and call for increased control (Quam 1990). According to Douglas (1966), any group that feels threatened tries to reinforce and control its boundaries and to create a dichotomy between the inside as healthy and the outside as polluted, thus drawing and creating a social analogy between pollution and disorder. In his iconography of disease, Gilman described how we define ourselves as safe and healthy by locating diseases elsewhere: "It is clear that we need to locate the origin of a disease, since its source, always distant from ourselves in the fantasy land of our fears, gives us assurance that we are not at fault, that we have been invaded from without, that we have been polluted by some external agent" (1988: 262).

The strength of the boundary drawn between the healthy and the polluted and the stigma associated with it is most strongly felt by the persons beyond that boundary, on the side of the polluted. HIV is unspeakable – at least beyond the circle of partners, friends, and family – to many of them:

> "HIV is tainted, isn't it. It seems not only to be a physiological state, it is something more, it is almost a social sickness. (…). I think in most groups you still can't talk about it. As an HIV-positive person I can't just talk about it in a group of people." (Peter Carreira)

> "People have a very different level of information and interest and deal very differently with HIV, and you never know how they deal with it. (…). I find that somehow annoying, that I can't simply say: I am HIV (sic[37]), and therefore I can't – I don't know, what is it that I can't?
>
> ck: Donate blood?
>
> Yes, exactly, for example. These verbal – how do you call that? – environmental, social, strange things are indeed the more difficult ones." (Andrea Meier)

> "This disease first appeared in a part of society people have huge problems accepting, which are the outsiders. First it was a gay disease, and then it was the junkies, that's just logic, it appeared wherever you had direct blood contact. In all social groups it was accepted as an outsider-disease, and that's what sticks in people's brains, that this disease is something special. But these people probably do not recognize that they are far off, that the virus caught all social strata throughout the world, throughout all structures, throughout all types of societies. But that it was at first a junkie-gay disease, that it appeared in the lower levels of society, that's in people's minds and you don't get it out of there anymore. Theoretically, it should be out, we call ourselves an enlightened population, (…), but that's not what we are." (Jakob Theiler)

---

[37] Also Salvatore Annoni used the formulation "I am HIV" (instead of the common "I am HIV-positive"). It may provide an example of a linguistic incorporation of the sickness, an extreme use of the "I am" reference to enduring sickness as it is exemplified by "I am an epileptic" or "I am schizophrenic" (Estroff 1993). "I am HIV" is a stronger joining of identity with diagnosis than the cited examples; its counter-piece would be "I am epilepsy" or "I am schizophrenia".

The strong perception of social stigma and exclusion stands in sharp contrast to the physical perception of the disease. People with HIV live with the paradox of a stigma brought about by a physical condition which they cannot perceive, with a sickness highly loaded with medical, social and cultural significance and yet without a physical presence. This duality of social existence/physical non-existence of the HIV infection ran through all the interviews with persons affected by the sickness, giving both the interviewees and myself the feeling of talking about "a shadow, or a ghost", "a chimerical state":

> "{HIV is} some invisible thing waiting someplace. I can't really judge it. Or, let's say, I can't foresee it. One of the things where you never know what will expect you. It is very difficult, I would say. It is here, it is present, and yet not, maybe like a shadow, or a ghost that keeps you company." (David Burki)

> "HIV is actually a chimerical state, it exists only in the labs and in people's minds, but it has so far not had any physical effect on my life. A social, a psychological effect, but no physical reaction. AIDS is much more concrete for me. That is maybe also a bit unfair, that we have to live with this state, this quasi-sick state as HIV-positive persons, that we are even classified as being sick through the insurance companies, that is a bit unfair, isn't it." (Peter Carreira)

> "{HIV means to me} everything and not much. When I forget that I am HIV (sic), I feel normal and healthy. When I get for example a flu, I think: Oh, there it is already." (Salvatore Annoni)

Similarly as their patients, physicians confronted with HIV also struggle with its hidden presence, its dual meaning of being both potentially deadly and yet an undefined "opponent". The ambiguity of HIV places the patient in an unclear position in regard to his/her main attribute within the health care setting, i.e. in regard to sickness. The patient is "sick and yet he is not", a situation that questions the "strategy" of the physician:

> "I think that {HIV} is actually a serious disease, a malignant disease, like the sword of Damocles above the person infected. He is sick and yet he is not, he is in a way in a different situation than someone having for example Leukemia or a cancer tumor. There the opponent is somehow more defined, and the strategy to fight it is clearer, too. The HI-Virus is insidious, undefined, and yet it mostly leads to death." (François Neher)

The shadow or ghost that accompanies people with HIV is capable of exerting a profound influence on their lives. As David Burki put it:

> "At that moment {when receiving a positive HIV test}, a world falls apart. But over the years I got the feeling that the cup that broke back then is being put together again, or it is being reconstructed."

The disruptive effect of sickness in a person's biography is especially pronounced when s/he receives the diagnosis of carrying a chronic or lethal condition. Corbin and Strauss (1987) described these conditions as separating the person of the present from the person of the past, thus disrupting the personal biography and creating the vital need to reconfigure it. They characterized biography through the three major dimensions: conceptions of self, biographical time, and body. Conceptions of self are continuous processes which are based upon experience. People therefore continuously adjust their conceptions of self while attempting to integrate various aspects of self into a whole. Conceptions of self differ in relation to the different situations in which people find themselves, and they change over biographical time. Biographical time is the constitutive aspect of biography, the core around which it evolves. As I will outline, it becomes highly uncertain with an HIV diagnosis. The body as the third major dimension of biography is, according to Corbin and Strauss, the medium by which conceptions of self are formed. It allows a person to take in and give off knowledge about the world, self, and others, it is the medium of communication, and it performs tasks associated with various aspects of self. For my work, I would like to complement the definition of the body given by Corbin and Strauss with Giddens' definition: "The body is not just a physical entity, which we 'possess', it is an action-system, a mode of praxis, and its practical immersion in the interactions of day-to-day life is an essential part of the sustaining of a coherent sense of self-identity" (Giddens 1991:81: 99). Giddens interpreted body awareness and regimes, including for example exercise and diet, as an expression of the construction and control of self-identity. The access to body regimes and health becomes one of the dominant focuses of class division[38]. Giddens thus described the body not only as a medium for human activity, but also as an outcome of this very activity (Shilling 1993).

In the following chapters 2.1. to 2.3., I will largely follow the three major dimensions of biography given by Corbin and Strauss – self, time, and body – to analyze how people confronted with HIV are trying to make sense of the infection and integrate it into the their lives. I am also expanding the approach of Corbin and Strauss by applying it to the constructions of HIV, of the person infected by it, and of the human body by people professionally confronted with the infection, i.e. physicians and scientists. In doing so, I aim at showing the mutual relationship between the perceptions developed by biomedicine and by people with HIV.

---

[38] The body as an expression of class-identity may also be reproduced by advertisements which create an analogy between human bodies and consumer goods: Stacey described how the body increasingly stands for the product to be sold and replaces it by taking on its qualities: "{T}here is a move away from an association of the product – say, a car – with romantic coupling and towards an increasingly isolated human figure. And that figure itself is as sleek and perfectly engineered as a really great car: The human body now has a kind of hard, metallic look to it" (Stacey 1999: 37).

## 2.1. SELF

The advent of chronic sickness marks, according to Bury (1982; 1991), a biographical disruption, the disruption of taken-for-granted assumptions by questioning the fabric of everyday life and the knowledge that underpins it. As the biographical continuity is ruptured, narratives "offer an opportunity to knit together the split ends of time" (Hydén 1997: 53). This knitting both relates the sickness to shared cultural assumptions and to moral causes hidden in our former lives. Stories about chronic sickness are thus not only descriptive, but also reflective by analyzing the events and reconfiguring knowledge and identity.

In our interviews, people with HIV commonly recounted their infection in opposition to Bury's concept of biographical disruption: Becoming infected is often less the cause for biographical disruption than the consequence of a personal crisis which is located *before* the infection took place and which caused the circumstances that favored an infection. The crisis is characterized by difficult social relations which join with a negative self-perception:

> ck: "You said somehow you were not surprised when you had your positive test?
>
> No, I wasn't surprised.
>
> ck: How come?
>
> Because I have been living miserably and living on the street and things like that.
>
> ck: So you expected it?
>
> That was sort of what I wanted, almost...
>
> ck: Why?
>
> That's how I am, I like to hurt myself and I used to be comfortable only when I was feeling bad. It was just another punishment that I wanted." (Eliane Dutoit)

> "Actually it was about time. I had many sexual partners, and when I look back now, I can't understand it, but it really was exaggerated. Something had to happen, and then I got this diagnosis and I felt: finally something happened." (Peter Carreira)

> "That I got infected through sex just seems logical to me now. I never took any responsibility with my first two partners, in terms of contraception, I was careless with my sexuality. Back then I was in an incredible crisis, actually for many years already, and nowadays I almost have to be grateful that this happened to me. I think I would not be the person I am now if that hadn't happened eleven years ago. It shook me out of my life and scared me to death, I can't put it any other way, I was really forced to look at myself. And that was my chance." (Jana Seifert)

Becoming infected is, at least in the narrative re-constructions, an almost desired climax of the times of crisis: "finally something happened". It is as if becoming infected is an embodiment of the crisis which was before only manifest in the social relations (Scheper-Hughes 1994). The virus transgressed the skin in social interactions – sex or needle sharing – to inscribe itself into the physical body. As the external is internalized, it also becomes materialized, testable, objective, and labeled, "HIV-positive".

This physical materialization is double-faced: On the one hand, it might help to reify the personal situation through an invading "it", a disease entering the body from the outside[39]. On the other hand, it carries the disorder formerly associated with the social situation to the inside of the body, thus creating new sites of uncertainty. According to Taussig, the social relations are thus mapped into the sickness. As he pointed out: "The attribution of disease to a foreign agent would seem as old as human-kind. But only with modern Western medicine and the late nineteenth century 'germ theory of disease' did this idea largely shed itself of the notion that the foreign agent was an expression of specific social relations" (1980: 246). As the example of HIV indicates, these different theories of sickness causation may easily live side by side.

It seems from the limited number of our interviews that viewing the infection as a biographical disruption, in accordance with Bury's model, is linked to a positive perception of the pre-HIV identity. David Burki described his life prior to the test and the circumstances of becoming infected as thoroughly positive, "we really lived back then, we had numerous adventures". The HIV test was a "big bang" for him, a world that was falling apart:

> "We really lived our lives. And that was the time when little by little the information came across, when little by little safer sex entered the discussion, and we started changing our behavior. But you have to see, back then we were let's say between 17 and 22, or 18 and 25 years old, and we really totally... – we went on vacation, abroad, had numerous adventures, we really lived back then, we did everything that was fun. And then that big bang. That's how I always say it. If the knowledge had been around five years earlier, or the virus had taken hold five years later, then maybe – and I must really say: maybe – it wouldn't have happened to us. When I look today at people I know who are five or ten years younger, most of them do not have these problems. But everybody else, or many I know of my age, born around 55, or 50 to 65, they really were totally in all that, when we lived and when, as it looks, the virus could spread easily. And, for heaven's sake, back then we lived, and we lived everything up, also our sexuality. (...). Back then I was around twenty, we traveled around, could travel, had the job, the money, traveled around, got to know a lot of people, did a lot of things, and that might have been the reason. That's how I look at it today."

Also in a physician's biography, diagnosing a person as HIV-positive may mark a decisive point. André Favre described his first encounter with his patient whom he subsequently tested seropositive:

---

[39] Cassell (1976a) described a linguistic distinction between diseases that are distanced and objectified as an invading and foreign "it", and others like diabetes and hypertension that do not seem to be referred to impersonally. He linked the presentation of disease as "it" to a culturally predominant objectified and depersonalized view of disease as an external thing invading the body, a view also represented by the germ theory.

"On May 2nd, 1989, I started to work as a general practitioner, and a week later, on
May 9th, I saw him for the first time. It is – it was an event that left its marks on me."

In an oral history of the memories of physicians who have cared for patients with
AIDS; Bayer and Oppenheimer compared physicians' narratives of their confrontation with AIDS with soldiers' war stories: "Their stories are like war stories shared
by soldiers throughout history, stories of individuals whose lives are transformed by
events beyond their control and who, in the context of such events, find their lives
enlarged and transformed by a historical moment none of them could have predicted" (1998: 1).

It is common amongst our interview partners with HIV to assume a high degree
of responsibility for their infection: The number of sexual partners was "exaggerated", sexuality was "careless", and "HIV was just another punishment that I
wanted". Eliane Dutoit described how the public view of HIV[40] as a sickness caused
by deviance influenced her personal view of HIV:

"When {AIDS} came, it was a big shock, it was something that only homosexuals had,
and therefore, the people were very much afraid, the life, way of living and everything
like that. It is true that it has that over it. That if you have AIDS, you didn't live your
life well... Which I agree with, in a sense, I still haven't gotten rid of that: (...) I just
haven't taken care of myself." (Eliane Dutoit)

Attributing responsibility for health and sickness to the individual corresponds to
a widespread view in the industrialized countries where it is often encouraged by
government health education. Describing sickness as the consequence of individual
carelessness applies especially to stigmatized conditions, including AIDS, and joins
with the attribution of blame (Helman 1994). The emphasis on individual
responsibility for health reflects a middle-class attitude toward health as a good that
must be achieved through self-control, an attitude that also mystifies the social production of disease (Crawford 1985). Following Weber (1993), Crawford interpreted
the concept of self-control as a central element of capitalist culture, an internalization of discipline. In the 19th century, self-control became the ideology of the rising
bourgeoisie which both guided its action and legitimized its privileges. The emphasis on self-control in the contemporary health discourse can be interpreted as an
expression of the importance of this value in capitalist culture: self-control "may
constitute the symbolic substance, the implicit meaning of the pursuit of health. It is
possible to say that health is thought about in terms of self-control. It is equally pos-

---

[40] The public discourse has been portrayed relatively early in the history of AIDS. See for example:
Albert (1986), Baker (1986), Clarke (1991), Jones (1992), Kirp and Bayer (1992), Köneke (1991),
Venrath (1994).

sible to say that the concept of self-control is 'thought' in terms of the medium of health" (Crawford 1985: 76-77)[41].

The individualizing view of the origins of infection is both integrated and contested by our interview partners. Moritz Pedrini whose narrative introduces the present part saw his infection as a consequence of having subjected himself and the largely hidden homosexual side of his sexuality to a social order which does not allow for deviance, and he thus described HIV as a "socially conditioned sickness, supported through the immunity reduction of oppressed people in an achievement-oriented world". The interpretation reminded me of a narrative, recounted by Williams, of a woman with arthritis who related her arthritis to "the stress perhaps of suppressing myself while I was a mother and wife" (1984: 188). Williams interpreted her history as an attempt to express the view "that illness arises out of our relationship to the social world, when personal identity and the social processes within which that identity is defined come into conflict" (ibid.: 192). This interpretation in turn evokes Herzlich's description of the social representation of health and illness as an expression of the individual's relationship with society. "Within this framework, the sick person is a symbolic figure: he is the exemplary victim of the forces bearing upon us" (1995: 162).

While taking responsibility for becoming infected may partly be an internalization of an individualized concept of health and sickness, it is also linked to claiming authority over the experience and control of the sickness. Taking over responsibility for health and trying to control it through deliberate action might receive central importance when facing a life-threatening and stigmatized sickness. As Lock (1993a) noted, in the face of independence as a high cultural value, loss of autonomy through sickness may produce contradictions in individual embodiment. Regaining autonomy towards HIV may thus reduce such contradictions. In a case study of a drug-using woman, Hassin (1994) showed that responsibility and control are central symbols of building up a new identity with HIV, an identity that contrasts the image of drug users as deviant and irresponsible. Responsibility and self-

---

[41] Self-control over health and sickness is measured through the Locus of Control Scales (Wallston 1978) that numerically express the extent to which people believe their health to be determined by their own action (internal control) or by external factors such as luck, chance, or powerful others (Pill and Stott 1982). The scale is inspired by the idea that attributing health to internal control is the desirable attitude of a responsible individual taking care of his/her health. A scale that builds upon the Locus of Control Scale is the Salience of Lifestyle Index which attempts to identify "those segments of a population most ready to alter their lifestyle" (Pill and Stott 1987: 132). Given the social and cultural history of the concept, it is hardly surprising that members of the lower classes were found to rely less on internal control and "thought they were only morally accountable {for their health} in very restricted circumstances" (Pill and Stott 1982: 43). Wrapping a middle-class morality of health as the result of individual responsibility into a scale will most likely produce the outcome that it is the lower class that does not live up to its standards, a finding that in turn helps to reconstruct class identity.

control as a key to living with HIV was highly pronounced by Simone Peyer. She described her life before becoming infected in negative terms. "I actually never really felt happy in my life, earlier", as she put it. In her retrospective account, she lacked self-respect and therefore was too careless in terms of choosing her partners, a carelessness that led to becoming infected. In contrast to the description of her former life, she characterized her new identity by her efforts to lead a responsible, self-determined life. Correspondingly, while not rejecting medical care and treatment in principle, she did not use any form of medical control of her HIV infection ("I take responsibility for that. It's not just a nonsense behavior of mine, it's concrete and conscious. I do that on purpose. And if the situation changed, I would have to admit, okay, it didn't work, now I need help, and I would accept this help"). She stressed self-determination in order to "feel happy, to a certain degree" as central factors for staying healthy, thus linking her ideas of the etiology of HIV to its control:

> "Well, I really try to think: what do I want to do with my life? (...) {I would like to} organize my life in a way that I feel happy, to a certain degree, although I certainly cannot always a hundred percent do what I like, there just are certain obligations everyone has. But I still believe to a certain degree I can control it quite well, and that might be a reason {for staying healthy}. It somehow gives me the feeling of control over my life, you know, not being subjected to all those influences always coming from everywhere, to how you learnt it, how you were raised, that it has to be that way until the end of life."

Taking stock of her experience with HIV, Simone Peyer ended our interview with the following conclusion:

> "In our system it is simply a fact that you do not take a lot of responsibility. I would find that to be important, that you look for yourself what you can do, what you can change, and that you actually do it."

Creating an identity as a person with HIV is a complex process which though does not necessarily take place. In a study amongst homosexual and hemophiliac men having a prolonged experience with HIV, Carricaburu and Pierret could, in contrast to their hypothesis, not observe the construction of a "positive illness identity". Rather than elaborating a positive identity around the infection, their interview partners reinforced their pre-HIV identity built around homosexuality and hemophilia (Bury 1982; Carricaburu and Pierret 1995). David Burki describing his pre-HIV identity as a young homosexual man in terms of freedom, adventure, traveling, having money, as cited above, might come closest to Carricaburu and Pierret's concept of biographical reinforcement.

To Jeff Dijon, becoming HIV-positive did not change his life. As he describes in more detail in the narrative introducing chapter 4, the crisis and disruption were postponed to the moment when his physician suggested he start taking treatment:

"The announcement that I should start taking treatment was worse than the announcement that I was HIV-positive. That was no problem at all for me, as if I had heard that
my hair started turning gray, it is strange. (...). {The announcement of treatment}
made me freak out because it brought me closer to the possible end, if there is an end
due to that. It meant becoming conscious of reality. When they tell you that you are
positive, there is no change in your life, that doesn't do anything, but when they tell
you that you have to take medication because you are seropositive, and otherwise
things will not go well, it is different. Yes, that is the moment to become conscious
that our chances diminish, and that is what is frightening, I think. (...). {When I
received my positive test}, I walked in there with a smile, and I walked out with the
same smile. It is strange."

In accordance with the minor effect that the infection had on his life, he does not
load it with significance. In the context of his life as a former drug user, the infection is one amongst other problems, "just another test in life". As he plainly stated:

"At the moment I have no explanation {for the infection}. It is shit, and that's it. A
sickness is just another test in life. I do not have anything more to say about HIV."

Frequent among our interview partners though was the construction of a positive
new identity with HIV, a process that is favored by the relatively stable course of the
infection in our study group. The new identity as a person with HIV provides an
inversion of the attributes of the pre-HIV identity. The old and the new identity are
constructed as counter-images, thus creating an opposition that might help to overcome the liminal situation after being tested HIV-positive. Within these processes,
the infection may be seen as a catalyst of change. This role may lead to a positive
estimation of the infection which might seem paradox at first sight. The inversion of
the negative aspects of the pre-HIV identity, brought about by processes of transformation which center around the culturally valued notions of self-control and
responsibility, thus provide a possible plot of the narrative reconstruction of the HIV
infection. In Good's (1994) adaptation of narrative theory, the plot gives order, an
underlying structure, a direction and meaning to a story, even if this meaning is
changing with time and the context of the recounting of the narrative. The plot
which describes HIV as a vector for positive change has most directly been
expressed by Moritz Pedrini:

"The HIV infection was certainly the most important and best thing happening to me
so far."

## 2.2. TIME

A central consequence of a positive HIV test is its influence on the projected biographical time. The new status means that decades of life expectancy might immediately be lost. For people having lived with HIV already since the 1980s, trying to
re-construct their biographical time is a highly complicated task. They had been
infected in a time when their physicians may have plainly predicted a life expectancy of a few years. Meanwhile, they have not only outlived their friends infected

around the same time, but also their life expectancy. Our interview partners therefore describe their relation with time as a process of struggling first to reduce their
projected biographical time and then, after having outlived it year by year, to re-
create their future already given up:

> "Back then there was still that row of three: Three years infected, three years sick,
> three years dead (sic). So I thought: Well, at the latest by then (numbering off the years
> at his fingers) I will be dead anyway." (David Burki)

> "According to the HIV center I should have been dead for six years now. In 87 I was
> informed about my HIV test, and back then they said: well, five years at the most. (…).
> I was convinced that I would not make it until 25, and if I'm lucky, I just about make
> it." (Jana Seifert who turned 30 the year before our interview)

> "I counted with two, three years. Back then, twelve years ago, they thought that the
> time of survival was three to five years. I even took a risk by opening up my own busi-
> ness because I thought: what can go wrong anyway, there is no time for anything to go
> wrong. (...) I planned my life as if it was short, just fun, fun, fun, and after some time I
> got really bored. (...). I have been feeling somehow in limbo for the last ten years. In
> the first two years it was fantastic, I felt so interesting. For the last ten years I have not
> been feeling any interesting at all anymore." (Peter Carreira)

The issue ultimately addressed in measuring biographical time is whether
HIV/AIDS is rather defined as a lethal or a chronic condition. In the memories of
people with HIV, encounters with physicians during the 1980s were often overshad-
owed by the prediction of death. Medical science and physicians started to describe
HIV as a potentially chronic and manageable, though ultimately lethal condition
towards the end of the 1980s (Herdt 1992; Treichler 1992). The shifting concept of
HIV from a lethal to a chronic infection is intimately tied to the introduction of antiretroviral treatment. The initial shift toward the chronic model was tied not only to
the insight that people infected were living longer than anticipated, but also to the
introduction of the first antiretroviral medication, AZT from *Burroughs-Wellcome*
(Fee and Krieger 1993a; 1993b). The more recent and much broader shift toward
chronicity began its onset in 1996 with the wide introduction of the protease inhibitors to complement the already used antiretroviral medication.

In the euphoria about the new combination therapies, the idea of HIV as a
chronic, medically manageable condition was established by comparing it with diabetes (and less prominently hypertension), an analogy initially brought forward at
the 1996 International Conference on AIDS[42]. The Swiss researcher Luc Perrin for
example was cited with this analogy, although using it with some precaution as a
future possibility still to be proven: "Although Perrin says he is dubious that complete eradication of the virus from the body will be possible[43], he holds out the

---

[42] As pointed out retrospectively by Richard Horton at the 12th World AIDS Conference (Rapporteur
Session "Clinical Science and Care", July 3rd, 1998)

[43] See chapter 2.3. for a discussion of the eradication theory.

greatest hope for people who have been recently infected. In such cases, Perrin suggests that after a heavy regimen of multidrug therapy for a year, one that includes a protease inhibitor, patients might be placed on a lighter regimen for the rest of their lives. Should this theory be borne out, Perrin says, HIV-positive patients may eventually be viewed much like people suffering from diabetes or hypertension" (Johnson 1997: 58)[44]. Such analogies should replace more common analogies to diseases perceived to be lethal, most prominently cancer ("with cancer, you die fast", as Salvatore Annoni said). Our data indicate that the comparison of HIV with diabetes was only partially convincing to people with HIV and general practitioners in our study.

*Table 8. HIV as comparable to diabetes or cancer (people with HIV)*

|  |  | n | % | Valid % |
|---|---|---|---|---|
| Valid | Diabetes | 15 | 32.6 | 35.7 |
|  | Cancer | 27 | 58.7 | 64.3 |
|  | Total | 42 | 91.3 | 100.0 |
| Missing |  | 4 | 8.7 |  |
| Total |  | 46 | 100.0 |  |

*Table 9. HIV as comparable to diabetes or cancer (general practitioners)*

|  |  | n | % | Valid % |
|---|---|---|---|---|
| Valid | Diabetes | 167 | 30.8 | 32.9 |
|  | Cancer | 340 | 62.7 | 67.1 |
|  | Total | 507 | 93.5 | 100.0 |
| Missing |  | 35 | 6.5 |  |
| Total |  | 542 | 100.0 |  |

As tables 8 and 9 indicate, about one third of both populations (35.7% of people with HIV and 32.9% of general practitioners) compared HIV to diabetes while the remaining believed cancer to be the better comparison. Perrin's doubtful hope that HIV-positive patients may eventually be viewed much like people suffering from diabetes or hypertension had not (yet) become the common view among people affected or general practitioners. This might reflect that the new image of HIV had only partially penetrated these communities, and it might foreshadow the increasing doubts, described in chapter 2.3., concerning the long-term controllability of the HIV-infection through early treatment.

---

[44] Copyright © 1997; Hillary Johnson; reproduced here by kind permission of the author.

The image of chronicity was not only introduced in reaction to changes in the therapeutic and thus epidemiological situation, but it was also actively created and diffused to alter the perception of the infection[45]. People with HIV, physicians, scientists and the pharmaceutical companies contributed to the image of chronicity for different reasons.

Physicians describe chronicity and the prolonged biographical time as a major argument to introduce the idea of treatment to their patients. Claude Keller for example believed that the image of HIV as a chronic sickness is a precondition to decide for treatment:

> (Before the patient started treatment) "I talked to him about his view of the sickness, what he expects of the future. The information and views he had were totally different from mine. He had a view of the 80s, of a progressive disease with death in the end. Now I am trying to pass to him the view of 96/97, which means, a chronic sickness with the need to take medication, but without deterioration. (...). I asked him what he expected of his future, if he had plans or not, and I realized that he shaped his ideas according to the people around him, the people he saw dying, other people in his milieu." (Claude Keller)

---

[45] The reciprocity of description and perception and the symbolic power of labels is also exemplified by the naming of HIV. The virus which was later described as causative agent of AIDS was discovered and named in 1983 and 1984 independently by three laboratories. How the "Retrovirus Study Group, which is empowered to rule on matters of retroviral nomenclature and classification under the aegis of a larger group known as the International Committee on the Taxonomy of Viruses" (Varmus 1989: 3) coined the name HIV, Human Immunodeficiency Virus, was described by Varmus, its chairman at that time. The description provides fascinating insight into the factors that entered the negotiations over the name. Most prominently, these negotiations included the expectations that the name would form a verdict over the fight for primacy of discovery between Gallo and Montagnier by choosing one of their names: "Some perceive, wrongly in my view, that our final recommendations will form a verdict upon contested issues of priority of discovery, issues that could influence patent rights, the awarding of major prizes, patriotic sentiments, and financial gains" (ibid.: 4). This verdict was omitted by explicitly stating that HIV was chosen in distinction to all existing names. As Varmus diplomatically commented: "A prolonged battle over the issue of a name for the AIDS virus is more than trivial because the battle may come – some might say it has come – to symbolize certain excesses of character for which scientists are often criticized" (ibid.: 8-9). While both Gallo and Montagnier belonged to the Study Group, Gallo declined to sign the agreement on the name "HIV", published in the journals *Nature* and *Science*. The second issue hotly debated was what kind of relation between the asymptomatic infection and symptomatic AIDS should be symbolized by the name. Varmus described clinicians' opinion on that question: "they were almost exactly divided over the issue of whether to exclude 'AIDS' from the name. Some took the position that patients would soon be fearful about any term that denoted the agent of AIDS as about a term that was explicit, a phenomenon our committee referred to as 'the evanescence of euphemism'. Others felt strongly that it would be easier to explain the difference between infection by the virus and the disease itself subsequently induced in a minority of infected people if the virus had a name with less pejorative potential" (ibid.: 6). The attitude of the committee on the issue is not only reflected in Varmus' description, but also by the fact that despite the clinicians being "almost exactly divided over the issue", the official agreement stated that the name "does not incorporate the term 'AIDS', which many clinicians urged us to avoid" (ibid.: 9).

The "view of 96/97" might indeed be a precondition to taking antiretroviral therapies. In our population of people with HIV, people who compared HIV to diabetes were significantly more likely to be taking antiretroviral therapies than people who compared it to cancer (p=0.019)[46], but it remains open if the image of chronicity was a precondition to or a consequence of taking treatment.

While physicians, as outlined in the following chapters of this book, have a variety of motives to favor or reject the idea of HIV as a chronic, medically controllable condition, the pharmaceutical companies profit from the image of chronicity. As Estroff (1993) argued for the case of schizophrenia, the growing number of and demand for jobs by mental health professionals contributed to defining the condition as chronic. In the case of HIV, the image of chronicity implies the extensive usage of expensive medication and laboratory tests as well as regular visits with the preferably specialized physician. *GlaxoWellcome's Combivir* for example, a combination of antiretroviral drugs, generated 454 million dollars in 1999 sales, 90% of which came from the United States and Europe[47]. In the perception of François Neher, shares are indeed the most reliable account of the efficiency of a drug:

> "As I say to my patients: if something really is a breakthrough, I do not have to study the latest scientific literature to find out about it. First the stock market finds out, the company that produces it, and when all of a sudden their shares are rising, then I know something is hot. I don't necessarily have to read the latest things all the times. And since the stock market of all these companies producing these triple combinations hasn't exploded because they found these wonderful products, I have the feeling that they are mediocre, not breakthrough drugs."

The profits of pharmaceutical companies through the marketing of antiretroviral drugs entered the broad discourse through the nearly impossible access of people living with HIV in developing countries due to their high costs (Hogg et al. 1998). In May 2000, the pharmaceutical companies *Boehringer-Ingelheim, Bristol-Myers Squibb, GlaxoWellcome, Merck Sharpe & Dome,* and *Hoffmann La Roche* announced a substantial price reduction for antiretroviral drugs in developing countries[48], but they were reluctant to say they would price drugs at cost, since doing so would reveal that profit, once research costs have been covered, can equal 90% of the prices charged[49]. By reducing prices due to public and political pressure, the

---

[46] Table not shown.

[47] http://www.hivnet.ch:8000/topics/treatment-access/, message no. 828, May 15th, 2000. In January 2000, I contacted one of the Swiss pharmaceutical companies in order to get an idea of their sales figures of antiretroviral drugs in Switzerland. After talking and exchanging emails with a very kind company representative, he finally wrote: "Congratulations to your successful and impressive study! After an internal investigation I unfortunately had to find out that it is not possible for me to communicate sales figures to the outside."

[48] http://www.hivnet.ch:8000/topics/treatment-access/, message no. 821, May 11th, 2000

[49] http://www.hivnet.ch:8000/topics/treatment-access/, message no. 822, May 12th, 2000

companies also aim at keeping their drug patents. Drug patent law was reinforced in the interest of pharmaceutical companies through the TRIPS agreement (Trade Related Aspects of Intellectual Property Rights) at the 1999 World Trade Organization meeting in Seattle (Editorial 1999; Pécoul et al. 1999) by setting minimum standards such as a 20-year patent protection. In cases of public health emergencies, countries are, according to TRIPS, allowed to make their own generic, cheap version of a drug after a payment to the pharmaceutical company holding the patent (compulsory licensing) and to import drugs from countries other than the country of manufacture (parallel importing). The examples of Thailand and South Africa though have shown that the United States limited these possibilities through trade and political pressure and thus bypassed TRIPS agreements to protect their drug companies (Boseley 1999; Wilson et al. 1999).

For people with HIV both in industrialized as well as in developing countries (Desclaux 1998), chronicity may provide a means to challenge the stigmatizing association of the infection with death and thus to describe HIV as a process with chances of intervention and reversion (Whittaker 1992). The hope that dissociating HIV from death might help to de-stigmatize the sickness was expressed by Eliane Dutoit and Simone Peyer, both living with HIV:

> "It {HIV/AIDS} has become a little bit, I would say, more accepted in society. The fact that it can be treated helps other people, allows them to think about it. It's a question of people not wanting to associate with this illness, and it allows them to live better with it. People are not confronted necessarily." (Eliane Dutoit)

> "In the beginning of course everybody was afraid. That's not surprising because we only heard: everybody dies from it. That's not so extreme anymore, but back then, it was somehow a death sentence, and that is what I was told. And everybody was trying to avoid the subject. (...). Now I feel that it goes more towards a chronic disease, with all these therapies, and I actually find that quite positive. I think that way it loses a bit that drastic effect of being lethal and all that." (Simone Peyer)

Chronicity stands for the gradual introduction of a "discourse of hope" into the HIV/AIDS discourse, a process that previously has been described for the discourse about cancer (DelVecchio Good et al. 1990). How forcefully the discourse of hope entered the AIDS discourse following the 1996 International Conference on AIDS may be illustrated by the cover page of an issue of the German magazine *Der Spiegel* from January 1997. It shows an AIDS ribbon whose color – red – has turned for the most part green to symbolize hope with the caption "The AIDS Wonder". The magazine article itself speaks of "the virus of hope going around" (Grolle 1997: 118). The importance of the 1996 Conference in the professional perception of HIV/AIDS was exemplified in a Dutch study where general practitioners most often attributed their positive change of attitude toward treatment to this conference (Redijk et al. 1999).

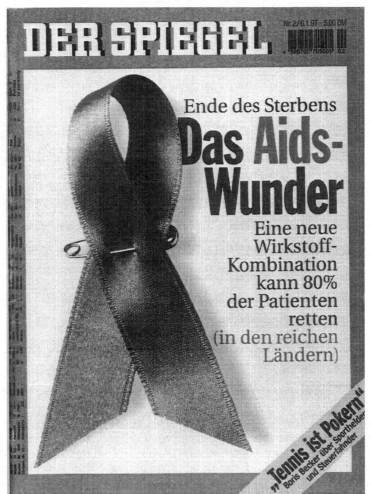

*Figure 1. The AIDS Wonder*
*Cover page of the magazine* Der Spiegel, *Issue 2, January 6, 1997.*
*Copyright © 1997;* Der Spiegel; *reproduced here by kind permission of* Der Spiegel.

The discourse of hope shifts the narrative biographical time of people with HIV from the immediate to the future (DelVecchio Good 1995b). Replacing what seemed to be certain death through an uncertain future does not only bring hope, but also emotional, practical and economic problems (Davies 1997). Long-term survivors addressed the "survivor's stress" of outliving one's friends (Pierce 1990) and being "sentenced to life" (Grimshaw 1994). The subject only entered the broad AIDS discourse when combination therapies started to prolong biographical time for a larger number of people with HIV and AIDS: "For several months the mainstream media have been full of anecdotal reports, many written in the first person[50], of people who were ready to cash in their life-insurance policies and quit their jobs in preparation for a round of high living before dying, but who now feel that their lives have been prolonged indefinitely" (Johnson 1997)[51]. Peter Carreira beautifully describes the uncertainties implied in the re-creation of biographical time:

> "Now I see the chance that I might after all still live for many years, even with strong medication that nevertheless offers an adequate quality of life. Of course, I did not expect that (laughs). I think this is why I have gradually revised a bit my whole attitude towards this sickness, towards *my* sickness. It is a glimmer of hope, although I of course do not look at it as a glimmer of hope because it actually turns my life upside down. Over the years I have so patiently come to terms with my days being numbered, and now I catch myself at thinking about my retirement: where do I want to retire? Here in Switzerland, or do I go back to my home country, or on some island? And so on and so forth. I catch myself at such thoughts. The question of pension fund; I have to deal with it, I can't just let it go. I am asked to take decisions."

## 2.3. BODY

Alice Theiler who had been infected through her husband described her reaction to the positive test:

> "I more or less broke down. I did not know what that virus does to me, or what happens to me inside of my body. My husband is in the situation that he lives long, that he lives and feels well. But how will my body react to this virus?"

What the virus does to the body and how the body reacts to the virus are central questions in HIV/AIDS research. The importance that scientists attribute to either the virus or the body, described as the "host", in determining the course of the infection runs along the lines of specialization. Virologists tend to focus their research and thus their explanatory models on the virus while immunologists stress the importance of the host's immune reaction. In the mid-1990s, both virologists and immunologists focused their research on HIV long-term survival and non-progression: The insight that some people with HIV have a more favorable course of the infection than others and possibly might never develop AIDS (Buchbinder et al. 1994; Easterbrook 1994; Schrager et al. 1994) led to the search for factors explaining the differences in disease progression. Implicitly or explicitly, this research was motivated by the hope of finding factors protecting long-term survivors or non-progressors against AIDS which can be converted into treatment of other people infected (Baltimore 1995).

---

[50] Also pharmaceutical companies use the emotional quality of first-person reports to represent the power of their medication. At the 1998 World AIDS Conference, I spoke to a man who traveled on behalf of *Merck Sharp & Dome* to conferences to tell the press about his new life through the protease inhibitor *Crixivan*. "I'm their Crixi man", as he put it.

[51] Copyright © 1997; Hillary Johnson; reproduced here by kind permission of the author.

In 1995, two articles in the *New England Journal of Medicine* set different accents in trying to find an answer to why some people had a more favorable course of HIV. The study group from the Laboratory of Immunoregulation and the Division of AIDS from the United States National Institutes of Health focused their research on the host's immune response in the lymph nodes (Pantaleo et al. 1995). The research group from the Aaron Diamond AIDS Research Center[52] in New York, a privately financed institute, set their main accent on virological factors (Cao et al. 1995)[53]. Although both research groups searched for viral as well as host factors and acknowledged that the two factors probably combine in determining the course of HIV, their exponents subsequently contributed to the polarization of the discussion. At the 1996 International Conference on AIDS, Giuseppe Pantaleo from the former research group and David Ho from the latter group became exponents of the host respectively the virus theory of HIV pathogenesis. The controversy over who could claim explanatory power over the HIV infection was carried out in the form of a plenary debate whose title already gave the answer to the question debated: "Pathogenesis: Resolved That Viral Factors, and Not Host Factors, Are the Primary Determinants of Pathogenesis"[54]. The debate, a powerful enactment of the verification of scientific theories through social activities (Fujimura and Chou 1994), culminated in Ho's conclusion: "It's the virus!". The conclusion elegantly took up Ho's position in an older debate on whether HIV is the cause of AIDS or not, a view that was most

---

[52] Following DelVecchio Good, the Aaron Diamond AIDS Research Center might be considered one of the globally leading "cultural centers of medical standard-making" (1995b: 469) in the field of HIV/AIDS.

[53] It is astonishing how the research groups seem to be composed along ethnic lines: The article by the Aaron Diamond research group with the Taiwan-born David Ho as their exponent is mainly authored by persons with Asian names while in the research group co-authoring with the Italian Giuseppe Pantaleo, a considerable number of Italian names appear. *Time* magazine explicitly linked Ho's history of immigration to his "extraordinary American success story" (Chua-Eoan 1996: 39), thus reconfirming the American myth. The article titled "The Tao of Ho" described the family's early years in a black community in central Los Angeles, Ho's difficulties of learning the new language and adapting to the new culture: "They were traveling to a land they did not know and whose language they did not speak. It would be a place where they would receive new names and new identities. Their father, a devout Christian, who now called himself Paul, had picked the boys' American names from the Bible. Thus it came to pass that Ho Da'i became David Ho and his younger brother became Phillip. For a few more years, Phillip would refer to David by the Chinese honorific for 'older brother'; becoming American would take time" (ibid.: 40). Nevertheless, becoming American was worth the trouble: "He plays down the importance of being Chinese to his success – but that is a very Chinese thing to do. Instead, he cites immigrant drive: 'People get to this new world, and they want to carve out their place in it. The result is dedication and a higher level of work ethic.' He adds, 'You always retain a bit of an underdog mentality.' And if they work assiduously and lie low long enough, even underdogs will have their way" (ibid.: 40).

[54] The debate stands in an old scientific tradition, as Mazumdar described it for the controversy about the nature of species fought amongst bacteriologists, immunologists, immunochemists, and blood group geneticists: "Their science was designed only in part to wrest an answer from *nature*. It was at least as important to wring an admission of defeat from their opponents — and these were opponents that never admitted defeat" (1995: 3).

prominently countered by Duesberg (1989). That debate had been clearly resolved in favor of the theory linking AIDS to HIV. As described in *Time* magazine, Ho "has been known to fling the occasional hot one-liner against naysayers – once 'It's the virus, stupid!' to those who insist HIV is not the cause of AIDS" (Chua-Eoan 1996: 39). Although Ho left out the "stupid" in the Vancouver debate, it inevitably rang in my ears.

Ho based his view that viral activity was central in determining the course of HIV on a study conducted by himself and colleagues showing that the plasma viremia quickly dropped in persons taking combination therapy (Ho et al. 1995). Based on this study, Ho and colleagues challenged the common view of asymptomatic HIV infection as an inactive phase by providing a model of "rapid turnover" or "viral kinetics". Given the rapid decline of plasma viremia, they assumed that the virus is highly active during the latency phase. In their description that quickly became the new paradigm, latency was now described as equilibrium between the production of millions of HIV particles and CD4 cells daily. As long as the CD4 cells can destroy as many virus particles as are produced, the equilibrium between the two antagonists is kept up and the amount of virus and CD4 cells remains stable – a stability characterized by constant action which Ho described through the metaphor of a runner on a treadmill. Only when the immune system cannot keep up the production of CD4 cells, viremia increases, the virus destroys more CD4 cells than the immune system produces, the number of CD4 cells decreases, and AIDS might develop. Or, in the more desired direction, when the virus replication is blocked through medication, as in the study by Ho and colleagues, the body's amount of CD4 quickly increases and viremia drops. According to Ho's description, the new paradigm could only be created through the availability of new techniques[55]: "In 1994 we had the techniques of measuring viral load very accurately, and we had the drugs {protease inhibitors} that would abruptly block virus replication efficiently – sort of put the brake on the treadmill. So we had a way of proving it – proving what the kinetic values are in HIV replication. And that was the paper published in *Nature*" (Johnson 1997: 53-54)[56].

In his often cited editorial from 1995, Ho called for "early aggressive treatment" of HIV, closing the editorial by stirring up hope that a cure for AIDS might be in

---

[55] Probably Ho was unaware of how nicely he illustrated the insight, brought about through social and cultural studies of science, that knowledge is partly shaped by techniques. As Rouse put it: "Scientific knowledge is often discussed as if it were a body of free-floating ideas detachable from the material and instrumental practices through which they were established and connected to things. Cultural studies (along with other recent studies of experimental practice) emphasize, instead, the importance of specific complexes of instruments and specialized materials, and the skills and techniques needed to utilize them, in shaping the sense and significance of knowledge" (1992: 11).

[56] Copyright © 1997; Hillary Johnson; reproduced here by kind permission of the author.

sight: "It was aggressive combination chemotherapy that led to cures {of tuberculosis and childhood leukemia}. Optimistically, we can hope that such an approach will become possible in patients infected with HIV-1" (1995: 450-451). Based on their short-term experiments with combination therapies, Ho and colleagues calculated in 1996 that virus eradication might be possible within 1.5 to 3 years of combination therapy (Perelson et al. 1996), an estimation prolonged by the same authors to 2.3 to 3.1 years in 1997 (Perelson et al. 1997). The spectacular claim for virus eradication brought Ho the title of *Time* magazine's 1996 "Man of the Year". One of the *Time* articles may illustrate to what extent science penetrates modern society: "Ho is not, to be sure, a household name – like Bill Clinton, who dominated the front page this year with his masterful comeback victory, or Bill Gates, who deftly extended the scope of his software empire into news, television and the Internet. But some people make headlines while others make history. And when the history of this era is written, it is likely that the men and women who turned the tide on AIDS will be seen as the true heroes of the age" (Elmer-Dewitt 1996: 29).

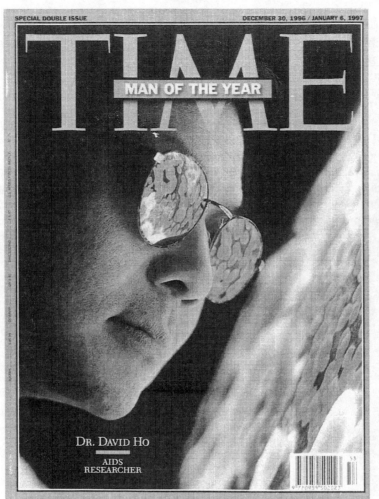

*Figure 2. Man of the Year*
*Cover page of* Time *magazine, Vol. 148. Issue 27, December 30, 1996 / January 6, 1997.*
*Copyright © 1996;* Time; *reproduced here by kind permission of* Time.

Ho's promise for eradication could not be fulfilled, but this only became apparent after his eloquent appearance already made him a star of science[57] and once more proved that, according to Koenig (1988), early reports of treatment success in

---

[57] Ho might have learnt for his public appearance, supported by a public relations firm (Johnson 1997), from the history of AIDS: "The study and attempts to control an AIDS 'epidemic' were thrust (by scientists) into the political arena where 'magic bullets' are sought and the most sensational claim is most likely to be quoted (i. e., the opposite of the 'organized skepticism' within science is what sells papers and rivets television viewers to their seats)" (Murray and Payne 1989: 123).

medicine tend to be rather uncritically accepted. Instead, less enthusiastic concepts entered the debate: The calculations concerning virus eradication did not include the notion that the virus may remain in body compartments referred to as "sanctuary sites" such as the brain beyond the reach of antiretroviral drugs (Cohen 1998)[58]. Ho's concept of rapid production of high amounts of virus was used to explain a rapid evolution of or even selection for virus types which are resistant to treatment (Condra and Emini 1997). Virus eradication remains incomplete with the given antiretroviral medication (Grossman et al. 1999; Young and Kuritzkes 1999), a fact also acknowledged in a more recent study by Ho and colleagues (Ramratnam et al. 2000). "Drug resistance", drug's "side effects" and "treatment failure" (Feinberg 1998) gradually became more popular rhetorical devices than "eradication" and "cure", ideas which were banned from the discourse.

The change in focus and explanatory power became most clearly enacted during the 1998 World AIDS Conference in Geneva. While Ho had dominated the 1996 Conference, immunologists gained territory in 1998. At the 12th World AIDS Conference in Geneva, Ho had to admit that he had overestimated the potency of antiretroviral therapies[59]. The immunologist Levy who had already earlier criticized Ho's concept was now in a position to say that the concept of virus eradication was naïve. With research underscoring the potential importance of the body's immune response, especially focussing on chemokines and their receptors, for the pathogenesis of HIV[60], immunologists claimed explanatory power. Levy emphasized the return of immunology by suggesting overcoming the polarizing discourse and bridging the gap between virology and immunology[61]. – As Oppenheimer concluded his review on scientific constructions of HIV already in 1992, "{t}he history of the epidemic demonstrates that the construction of HIV is a dynamic process in which different scientific specialties negotiated definitions that, to a degree, reflected their relative power" (1992: 75).

---

[58] The article by Cohen reporting a scientific meeting provides a rich example for the use of metaphors in medical science: "an ocean of HIV in patients" – "the immune system's radar" – "enlist the immune system" – "sanctuary site" (ibid.: 1854-1855).

[59] "Turnover of HIV", Oral Session "Viral and Cellular Dynamics", June 30, 1998

[60] For a review, see Lee and Montaner (1999). Chemokine immunobiology is, as I argue elsewhere (Kopp 2002), the site where new risk categories and risk groups are currently being created.

[61] Levy made both statements cited during the "Rapporteur Session, Track A: Basic Science", July 3rd, 1998. The Rapporteur Session is a conclusion and summary of the whole conference which is divided into four main subjects, referred to by "Tracks". The alphabetical order represents importance and prestige of the Tracks: A is "Basic Science", B "Clinical Science and Care", C "Epidemiology, Prevention and Public Health", and D "Social and Behavioural Science". Track D was only introduced in 1989. The fact that it was an immunologist reporting on Track A in 1998 again indicates how immunology regained territory. In 1996 however, it was Deborah Birx, director of the Division of Retrovirology of the Walter Reed Army Institute of Research (http://wrair-www.army.mil/cgi-bin/retrovirology-phone.idc), who reported on Track A.

The distinction between virology and immunology is also expressed through the metaphors that scientist from the two disciplines use to describe their approaches. Possibly the most prominent and widely cited metaphor in HIV research during the last years was – of course – coined by David Ho[62]. He titled the editorial in which he argued for starting therapy early in the course of the infection and with a combination of different agents with: "Time to Hit HIV, Early and Hard" (1995). In accordance with the title, he described antiretroviral treatment as "a number of better weapons with which to fight HIV-1" and called for "early aggressive treatment" (ibid.: 451). Since Ho could neither keep the promise of virus eradication nor is AIDS by now curable, as he hoped in his editorial, one may wonder if he might have used war metaphors for the purpose that Logan and Scott attribute to them, namely obscuring uncertainty: "At a more basic emotional level, the use of metaphor, especially military, has obscured uncertainty and powerfully influenced medical practice and policy making" (1996: 596).

War metaphors are a commonplace in medicine (Annas 1995; Wilson Ross 1989). The war metaphor emphasizes the virologist's view of HIV/AIDS as a disease determined mainly by the action of the virus, an outside invader, an aggressor to be treated aggressively. Ho reproduces a concept of disease which is predominant in American medicine: "Viruses, and by extension antiviral drugs, stand for external origins of disease in American biomedical discourse" (Feldman 1995: 101). This discourse tends to overemphasize external agents while neglecting the role of the "terrain", the host. Aggressiveness, directed against the external agent, is the key term to describe treatment (Payer 1988). It is only through such a focused view that the hope for a "magic bullet", a single drug that cures the infection, can be sustained. Similarly, metaphors of war and aggression depend on models of disease focusing on external agents. Describing both the infection as well as its treatment as weapons invading the body runs the risk of creating an analogy between these two antagonistic forces. The analogy may be illustrated by the use of the "bomb" metaphor in our interviews. While André Favre described the outbreak of AIDS as a "bomb going off", Marco Deville saw combination therapy as a "tremendous bomb" eradicating the virus inside the body:

> "And then there is this time bomb phenomenon. (…). When AIDS starts, the train has gone, you can rather precisely estimate the course. (…). When the bomb goes off, it is too late." (André Favre)

> "That's what the Americans are doing nowadays: Put a tremendous bomb inside to eradicate it as long as it hasn't happened yet." (Marco Deville)

War metaphors are used also in medical imagery and terminology to describe both the HIV infection as well as biotechnology developed to fight against it. In the

---

[62] As Johnson remarked, Ho "seems to revel in creating simple, powerful metaphors that annoy his scientific brethren but are eagerly embraced by laymen" (1997: 53).

advertisement for a book on AIDS entitled "AIDS Understanding Molecular Biology: The Invaders Are Here! A Unique Story", the two HI-Viruses George and Eddy invade the body from a "far corner of the universe called Monkeyland"[63].

---

[63] According to Haraway (1989), the equation of outer space and the inner body is common in the imagery of the body.

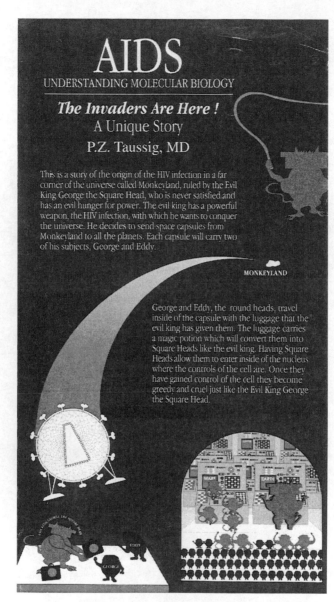

*Figure 3. The Invaders Are Here!*
*Advertisement for the book "AIDS Understanding Molecular Biology: The Invaders Are Here! A Unique Story" by P.Z. Taussig,* Doctors Press Inc., *1996.*
*Copyright © 1996;* Doctors Press Inc.; *reproduced here by kind permission of* Doctors Press Inc..

The image of biotechnology as armed aggression towards the virus is taken up, although played down in the image of a shooting gallery, by a firm that sells a system for HIV genotyping. HIV is presented as a "Moving target", but contrary to Ho's vision of antiretroviral treatment as a weapon to fight HIV, the "sure hit" in this case only refers to accurately counting the virus, not to killing it.

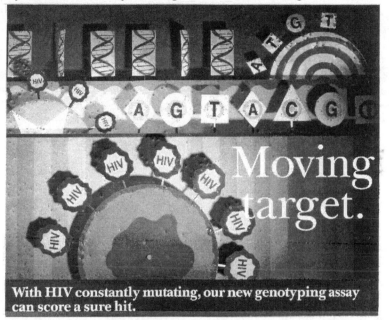

*Figure 4. Moving target*
*Invitation by the company* PE Biosystems *to a meeting entitled: "Developing an Integrated System for Sequencing-Based HIV Genotyping", 12th World AIDS Conference, Geneva, June 30th, 1998.*
*Copyright © 1998;* Applied Biosystems; *reproduced here by kind permission of* Applied Biosystems.

Using a similar type of terminology, the company *Vertex Pharmaceuticals* describes its dedicated "crusade" against the virus which again appears as a "ticking bomb" within the body: "The virus is a constantly moving target, a ticking bomb whose timer is set differently in every person. When attacked, it reinvents itself. It assaults the body's defenses, then invites other diseases. In the crusade to develop new AIDS medications, there is no room for complacency. Lives are at stake. We do not have a moment to lose."[64]

---

[64] Advertisement text by *Vertex Pharmaceuticals Incorporated*, published in: *a&u America's AIDS Magazine*, Vol. 7, Issue 45, no. 7, July 1998, p. 27. Copyright © 1998; *Vertex Pharmaceuticals Incorporated*; reproduced here by kind permission of *Vertex Pharmaceuticals Incorporated*.

As Patton pointed out, "virology and immunology can be viewed as new articulations of more longstanding models" (1990: 58). While virology stands for sickness as caused by external agents, immunology locates health in internal dynamics. Contrary to virology, immunology has largely moved away from the military metaphors, a move that was interpreted by Haraway (1989) as crucial for its current high theoretical status within science and society. The power of immunology in creating and defining knowledge is also reflected in the economic value of its object, the immune system. Supporting research into the immune system, although complex and difficult to access, is presented as a strategy of survival for pharmaceutical companies: "To survive in the future, drug companies are having to seek out drug targets in less accessible, more complex biological systems, such as the brain and the immune system" (Abbott 1993: 765). Likewise, for philanthropic foundations which are trying to "maximize the value of their funds", immunology ranges among the "hottest new fields": "most {philanthropic foundations} try to maximize the value of their funds by concentrating on new fields that they feel deserve particular attention for limited periods of time. Currently, the hottest among these are genetic research, neuroscience, molecular biology, immunology, AIDS, breast cancer and women's health, ageing and preventive medicine" (Greene 1993: 742).

Haraway described a gradual shift from viewing the immune system as a hierarchically and centrally organized system toward a "fluid and dispersed command-control-intelligence network" (1989: 12). Martin (1994) showed that along with giving up hierarchical ranking, nationhood and military metaphor, and rigid self-nonself distinction, immunologists increasingly constructed the immune system as a network of communicating cells that learn and adapt and thus combine specificity with flexibility. She linked the contemporary emphasis on the immune system and the emergence of an image of a non-hierarchical, flexible system to a change in capitalist production from Fordist hierarchically organized, factory-based production to contemporary flexible accumulation described through constant innovation and flexible response to new markets. The new image of the immune system is thus an embodiment of flexible accumulation. Immunologists are therefore not only creating knowledge to be dispersed into the outside world, but they also take up outside changes to be integrated into their production of knowledge. Martin hypothesized that immunologist might be more flexible than other scientists partly due to the fast changes brought about by AIDS research.

Her hypothesis seems to be confirmed through new research into genetic susceptibility for HIV infection and progression. The description of the immune system that Lee and Montaner gave in a 1999 review article of chemokine immunobiology in HIV pathogenesis evoke what Martin and Haraway described as the postmodern, late capitalist image of the immune system: "It has become increasingly apparent that the immune system maintains a delicate balance between the positive and nega-

tive regulators that govern the chemokine and cytokine networks" (Lee and Montaner 1999: 552). The metaphors of "delicate balance" and "network" imply constant
activity without hierarchy and aggression. Remarkably, this image is visually
emphasized in a figure which shows the immune responses to HIV in the shape of
the *yin-yang,* thus supporting Martin's hypothesis that imagery from the alternative
health discourse seems to become more relevant to the scientific description of the
body (Martin 1996a; 1997). Lee and Montaner described the *yin-yang* figure as
follows: "Hypothetical balance between the viral inductive and suppressive activity
of type 1/type 2 immune responses is illustrated by the Chinese concept of *yin-yang*:
that positive and negative forces are always in counterbalance" (1999: 559).

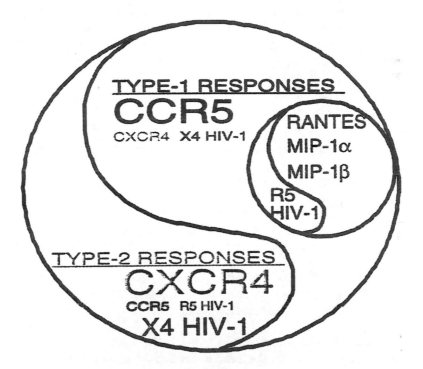

*Figure 5. Positive and negative forces are always in counterbalance*
*Lee and Montaner (1999: 559, Fig. 3).*
*Copyright © 1999;* Society for Leukocyte Biology; *reproduced here by kind permission of*
*the* Society for Leukocyte Biology.

The metaphors contradicting the non-hierarchical image are the "regulators" that
"govern" the network. Such metaphors of regulation and government refer to the

"old" image of the body and the immune system organized around hierarchy, war-
fare, and nationhood. With such an old image of HIV in mind, Lee and Montaner
finished their review by respectfully referring to the virus as the immune system's
(or, as the reader wonders, the researcher's?) "formidable enemy". They hoped that
further research "will help increase our understanding of how the immune system
functions in the vise of such a formidable enemy as HIV" (ibid.: 560). As Martin
(1992b) pointed out, the two images are theoretically contradictory. In practice,
these contradictions reflect "the world outside the body" where localism, nation-
alism, and class division have not only remained, but partly also been reinforced
under the global economic system.

The image of a delicate balance between the virus and the body largely corresponds to how people with HIV describe their infection. They refuse to declare their
own bodies as battleground by developing a counter-discourse of a peaceful integration of the virus and the body. David Burki for example described his relation
with the virus in the following words:

> "I simply have the feeling that when I look well to myself and when I feel well, then
> maybe for that reason the virus keeps quiet or something."

War metaphors were also challenged by creating new meanings of the abbreviation "AIDS". They provide alternative ways of preventing AIDS which are opposed
to aggressive approaches. One person edited a journal named "Angst In Dir Selbst"
(Fear Inside Yourself). In an article entitled "Fear Is the Killer", he described fear as
the real social syndrome, more common and more problematic than AIDS, since it
causes more people not to live their lives than AIDS does. The negative effect of
fear is especially pronounced in AIDS patients, and the adequate alternative to it is
the alliance with "love and life": "There are probably many more people getting sick
in soul or body from fear of AIDS than there are AIDS patients. Fear itself turns into
a risk behavior. (...). Especially in AIDS patients we see how fear can paralyze all
processes of life. (...). What we can do is to form an alliance with the contrary of
fear, with love and life" (Arbeitskreis HIV 1996: 17).

Jana Seifert re-interpreted "AIDS" as "Alles In Dir Spürt" (Everything inside of
you feels), and the feeling that she learnt to develop through the confrontation with
the infection was also her prophylaxis against developing AIDS:

> "Everything inside of you feels, that is what AIDS means to me, and that is my
> prophylaxis, my way."

The two alternative interpretations of AIDS are thus linked to alternative treatment approaches, or an alternative "prophylaxis", as Jana Seifert put it, which is
encoded in the language. In both examples, the factors that cause or inhibit AIDS
are located not in the virus, but in the person confronted with the infection, a construction that helps to adhere to the notion of controlling the infection. Simone

Peyer even explicitly argued against theories emphasizing the virus as determining the course of HIV:

> "I have the feeling (...) that a human being is more than a virus. I think, the danger is that everything is seen to depend on the virus. I have the impression that you can do much more with your lifestyle and your attitudes."

Models of disease progression that emphasize the virus as the main or only factor were commonly rejected by our interview partners with HIV for two main reasons: Firstly, they are too normative as the individual in his/her uniqueness is bracketed out in explaining the course of the infection (Champaloux 1996). Secondly, they do not allow for the possibility of control by actively influencing the infection through lifestyle and attitude, as mentioned above by Simone Peyer. The belief in a multi-factorial model of disease progression, which includes elements that are potentially controllable by the person infected, was also reflected in the questionnaire survey.

Table 10. Perceived influence on the course of HIV (people with HIV)

|  | n | % |
| --- | --- | --- |
| Psychic attitude | 36 | 80.0 |
| Medical treatment | 27 | 60.0 |
| Lifestyle factors | 27 | 60.0 |
| Biological factors | 36 | 80.0 |
| Other factors | 9 | 20.0 |
| No factors |  |  |
| Don't know | 4 | 4.4 |
| Total | 45 | 100.0 |

Among people with HIV, all the four factors asked for were believed to influence the course of the infection by a majority of the study group. Most frequently named were attitude and biological factors[65] (80% each), followed by medical treatment and lifestyle factors (60.0% each). Such a multi-factorial model of disease progression, including also attitude and lifestyle, was common amongst physicians as well. André Favre for example adhered to it to explain an unexpected course of HIV in his patient:

> "The Federal Office of Public Health gave out recommendations – a long time ago, of course, maybe five, six, maybe even a bit longer, seven years ago – on behavior. Balanced nutrition, always being physically active but without exaggerating it, taking breaks, enough sleep, enough rest, trying to omit severe stress. Well, I believe that these are plausible possibilities. I mean, there must be something about it. My patient

---

[65] Biological factors were defined in the questionnaire as "the body's defences, type of virus, general health status". In writing this book, I regret that we did not ask about body's defences and type of virus in two separate questions.

has a severe infection, it's not like he had only slightly been positive, rather he was flooded with this virus. In that sense, he certainly had a bad precondition, had lymph nodes from the first moment on. And now, eight years later, he is still somehow, as it looks to me, in category A or what they call it nowadays, that means he has no clear infections. (…). I believe his lifestyle did contribute to that." (André Favre)

*Table 11. Perceived influence on the course of HIV (general practitioners)*

|                    | n   | %     |
|--------------------|-----|-------|
| Psychic attitude   | 342 | 65.1  |
| Medical treatment  | 479 | 91.2  |
| Lifestyle factors  | 303 | 57.7  |
| Biological factors | 458 | 87.2  |
| Other factors      | 80  | 15.2  |
| No factors         |     |       |
| Don't know         | 30  | 5.7   |
| Total              | 525 | 100.0 |

A majority of general practitioners believed that medical treatment (91.2%) and biological factors (87.2%) influenced disease progression. Similarly though as people with HIV, a majority of general practitioners also believed in attitude (65.1%) and in lifestyle (57.7%) as influencing the course of HIV. People with HIV as well as general practitioners thus tended to reject a mono-causal model and also expressed their belief in individual and potentially controllable factors as influencing disease progression. In accordance with this multi-causal model, a vast majority of the study population of people with HIV had already changed elements of their lifestyle, most notably elements of their diet[66] (Kopp et al. 1999).

The interface mediating lifestyle and attitude into health is the immune system. The image of the immune system as a flexible network that constantly learns and adapts is logically linked to the idea that it can also be trained (Haraway 1989; Mar-

---

[66] This emphasis on diet might not be surprising, given that, according to Turner, diet represents an attempt to organize the body both in religion and medicine: "It has been suggested that diet in a religious framework is the management of the interior body while in a secular medical practice, it becomes increasingly the organization of the exterior body in the interest of longevity and sexuality" (1995: 26). As Helman (1994) pointed out, moral concerns are increasingly being expressed in medical, rather than religious terms, and religious ides of sin and immortality may become replaced by ideas about sickness and health. Where religion speaks out against a "sinful life", medicine condemns an "unhealthy lifestyle", with a main difference that the punishment for the unhealthy lifestyle or the reward for the healthy lifestyle is not delayed to the world to come, but occurs in this world. The association between religion and medicine became most apparent to me when I worked as a counsellor for anonymous HIV testing. People talking, liberated through the medical obligation for openness and the anonymous setting, about their sexual life, often evoked to me the setting of the catholic confession I am familiar with from my catholic upbringing.

tin 1994). As Illich put it: "Nowadays a human who seeks health is according to common sense a subsystem of the biosphere, an immune system to be controlled, ruled, and optimized as 'a life'" (1999: 3). The immune system as an adaptive and trainable system central to our healthy self has become such a common image that it is difficult to keep in mind that it existed as an explanatory category for only a rather short time: Martin (1990) points out that it was only in the mid-1960s that macrophages, lymphocytes, and other cells came to be seen as part of a mutually interacting body system, the immune system. Only in the 1970s departments of immunology were founded in universities, and popular ideas of the immune system grew frequent as late as in the 1980s. The idea of the immune system not only as a personal disposition for health, but also as an adaptive system to be shaped and worked out was expressed by some of our interview partners:

> "I have right away excluded the possibility of early intervention because I never perceived that to be important, I never thought that might be good. Even before, as a child, I was educated that way. Rather hostile against doctors, if you want to put it in a nasty way, and that certainly contributed to my attitude. We did not always run to the doctor. (…). For that reason I somehow developed a better self-perception than if I had always taken antibiotics right away. We really only rarely took strong medication and I just have the feeling that it is even another reason why my immune system is somehow stronger than when somebody always takes strong medication for the smallest problem. That's why I rely on my immune system, I simply have the feeling that it is strong." (Simone Peyer)

> "I am convinced that every disease I go through strengthens my immune system. It just takes its time. (…). I just know how many destructive things I shot into myself, into my body, and based on that I just have to say that I obviously have a strong immune system, or I would not be so healthy today. (…) I do care for myself, nutrition is something important to me. Cooking is also my hobby, I am fortunate for that. Therefore I love being a creative cook. And I do a bit of sports, at least once a week. Or meeting with friends. All these things are good for me, and they are certainly also good for my immune system." (Jana Seifert)

Simone Peyer and Jana Seifert refer to popular ideas of the immune system, as expressed for example in an article entitled "Strengthen Your Immune System", published in a journal available in Swiss pharmacies: "A healthy lifestyle, balanced nutrition, and natural prevention strengthen the immune system and put an end to viruses and bacteria" (Dürst 1999: 37). Simone Peyer's belief that reluctance in consuming strong medication, namely antibiotics, corresponds to the quote attributed to a professor Jean-Michel Dayer that closes the article: "'Too early preventive interventions confuse the body's sensitivity and hinder its alarm function. As this century comes to an end, we probably face the danger of exaggerated prevention instead of letting ourselves be guided by our own alarm signals'" (ibid.: 39).

Jana Seifert creates an implicit analogy between HIV and her former drug use: drugs were also entering her body, or actively brought into her body by herself, as destructive agents, but they ultimately could not harm herself due to the strength of her immune system. Crawford (1985) described HIV as a "Trojan horse", shifting danger to the inside of the body. In the face of the virus already having entered the body, the body's boundary is not valid as protective layer between self and other anymore. Strength expressed through the immune system locates protection within the body to combine the danger of the virus inside the body with the ability to remain healthy.

With boundaries between self and other relocated to the inside of the body, the body becomes increasingly uncertain and fragmented. As our bodies are populated by invaders from without, they cannot be viewed as coherent units anymore. Coherence is pushed back to the boundaries of the body's parts that receive a life of their own. The physician Franz Jann described how his patients tended to define their CD4 cells as persons populating them:

> "Many sick people also have a very paradox relationship with their CD4 cells. When you tell someone for example: now you have eight CD4 cells left, then he says: now Edi has died. And then you ask: who is Edi? Well, that was the ninth. Stuff like that. That they give names to their CD4 cells is very common. When they are really below ten, then they quasi get names, the CD4 cells. To us that is ridiculous because it can change from one moment to the other according to how many lymphocytes you get. But the number on the paper receives a very important status. For which, of course, if you want to put it that way, we are to blame, too, as we are so preoccupied with the CD4 cells." (Franz Jann)

Patients' views are often described in exotic terms in physicians' "storytelling" (Mattingly 1998), as represented in the above case through adjectives like "paradox" and "ridiculous". Such attributes help to distance the patients' views and to shape them into beliefs, as opposed to medical knowledge. Yet despite being "ridiculous", Franz Jann presents the importance attributed to the number of CD4 cells also as a direct consequence of the view that physicians "so preoccupied with the CD4 cells" carry into the health care process. Not only the preoccupation with, but also the personalization of cells is common in biomedicine, as vividly shown for example by Haraway (1989: 27) for the case of the immune system. Referring to scientific and popular images attributing personhood to human cells, Martin suggested: "It is possible that in the 1990s what was the patient (or person) has itself begun to become *an environment* for a new core self, which exists at the cellular level" (1992a: 415, emphasis in original). While human cells are presently still valid entities in the AIDS discourse, they in turn already have been fragmented by science. As genetic research has disassembled the cell and as the body's protection against HIV is relocated to the genetic level of the immune system ("Resistance to HIV-1 Infection: It's in the Genes"[67]), it is possible that the boundaries of the new core self might eventually be pushed back from the cellular to the genetic level.

---

[67] As Fauci (1996) entitled his discussion of recent research. See also Kopp (2002) on the construction of HIV/AIDS risk.

# CHAPTER 3

# TRANSLATING MEDICINE TO ORDINARY PEOPLE

> "Cautious skepticism is simply what any sensible person is inclined to exercise when dealing with professionals who have the kind of power that doctors have over their patients' lives."
> (Durant 1995)

## ANDREA MEIER: A BALANCING ACT

For the first time now I was really profoundly moved by this treatment decision. So far I always thought: I feel well, and that's the most important, I feel well now, and I don't think that far into the future, and the past, that's over, I can't change that anymore, it is how it is. And a treatment decision is always oriented toward the future, you start planning: What could happen? That really got me, really for the first time, how shall I say, almost pulled me down, because there are all these abstract figures, CD4 figures and viremia and tablets, so many tablets, and traveling so many times to the HIV center, and I might not get anything out of it. Maybe, maybe not. And then I thought that somehow this is much worse for me than when I just think: I am feeling well, and maybe I do not know too much. In addition, I planned to go hiking in France and to take a language course in Spain this summer, and then I just do not want to organize my whole life around this medication. For I see that somehow I would place my hopes too much on the medication instead of on myself, and for the moment that's an imbalance to me. That's why I now just thought: not for the moment, in fall I might think about it again.

Actually it was good now to really think about it, because it did indeed get closer again. Also with all these people – family and friends – around me. I intensely talked to some twelve people about it, just to hear how others would deal with something like that, how they see it. That was a good thing, also just to know that all these people are around, no matter what happens. And that was actually what was good for me, this very basic reflection: What is the matter with my life? What will I still do and what do I want now?

I thought for a long time about going into psychiatric treatment. I mean, treatment, just talk to someone, since I was confronted with so much, and all these people that know me, they are emotionally affected, want the best for me and don't really know either. And it was a big thing in my family, and so I thought, somehow I should talk to someone not so involved, who can speak objectively. I had already looked for addresses,

50

but then I dropped it again. I also contacted physicians, called the "Aids-Hilfe", all the things that I had never done before, looked everywhere for information, and everybody was a bit at their limits. My general practitioner was helpful, he could really tell me that there were so and so many tablets, and different complicated combinations, these tablets in the morning, these at noon, these in the afternoon, and that was what I had to expect. I think that's very good about him, he doesn't just say: now you have to, and do this, and watch out. Instead, he really tries to tell me as he knows me I have been rather cautious about medication and always tried it with nutrition and things like that, and therefore he would suggest to think it over. I just prefer this way to someone trying to put pressure on me, saying: now you have to. Because then I don't understand why I do something, whose opinion it is. As far as I am concerned, a physician doesn't have to tell me what I have to do, he has to inform me. Although, it actually means more than providing information, it also means, somehow, translating medicine to ordinary people. We somehow have a relationship that made me realize he is interested as well, and he passes on what he knows, and that's quite good.

I have been with him since, yes, since 89. I went there as I suspected – well, it was a complicated story – as I suspected that I might have been infected. He has been in-volved in my care since the very beginning. And he also knows my partner, and all these conversations are always quite personal. When I just used to go there once a year to be monitored, I found that it was of no use for me, and he didn't know anything more to do (laughs). Then I thought that I might have to talk to someone who is less concerned with the medical side of it. But now I have given up that idea, since now, somehow, I found that medicine is again an issue now, and you can't neglect that any-more, nowadays. I mean, I can't just go into the woods and say goodbye, I have noth-ing to do with the world anymore. That's why I think it is good for me now.

Back then, when I went less to the physician, laboratory values didn't mean anything to me, I didn't want to know how many cells and things like that, because it didn't mean anything to me. Although now, with the perspective of medication, laboratory values are, yes, important. You are almost a bit forced to it. Except if you were just to say no to everything, that of course is another possibility. I'm of course always a bit in conflict, I also always think: in earlier times, it was like this or like that, but I mean, we live now, in 1997, and science and medicine came to this point, and we are all in-volved in it, in one way or another. You can't just say no to everything, because then you can't live in this world anymore. Somehow it is also a way of being realistic, with these laboratory values. If indeed these CD4 values were dropping now, then I cer-tainly would try it with these drugs, there somehow is a glimmer of hope, that's clear. I somehow just thought that I will still wait a bit, and I just monitor it more regularly. It is after all a balancing act, because you should not wait until they really drop, then it is simply too late. It is not easy if you have to make these decisions that suddenly give you the feeling: you might fall ill. Death might be close.

***

The introduction of combination therapies profoundly influenced the interaction between patients and their doctors. As a consequence of medical powerlessness and active involvement and interference of persons afflicted, the early phase of the HIV epidemic was characterized by new approaches to public health. They included a major emphasis on prevention[68] and privacy rights, and collaboration between people affected, social movements, public health officials, medical professionals, and political parties. These approaches are commonly described as "HIV exceptionalism" (Bayer 1991; Rosenbrock et al. 2000). The state of exceptionalism also left its traces on the doctor-patient interaction. In the situation of medical impotence, physicians who had to offer little in the face of a deadly disease were confronted with well-informed and active patients, above all gay men. While activism tended to empower patients, the relative inability to act tended to reduce physicians' authority since "{i}n the absence of medical power, it was difficult to be arrogant" (Bayer and Oppenheimer 1998: 5). To some degree, the combination of bottom-up activism and therapeutic impotence leveled off the inequalities inherent to the doctor-patient interaction and entailed what Bayer called "a new, more 'democratic' style of medicine" (ibid.: 5).

The "patient as expert" became a key rhetoric to grasp the new doctor-patient interaction: "In this sense, the doctor-patient relationship is not a simple relationship between an expert and a relatively uninformed layperson but, in a real sense, a meeting between experts" (Walker and Waddington 1991: 129). André Favre similarly described the relation with his patient as actually dissolving the doctor-patient relationship (which is therefore implicitly described as being asymmetric by definition) by being an exchange on an equal level. In his description, though, such an interaction is not characteristic for all encounters with HIV patients:

> "He always challenged me, in a pleasant way. He was always up to date, sent me sometimes articles to have a closer look at something (...). With him, it is indeed closer than with other {HIV patients}. That somebody knows so much about it – he actually knows more than I do – does not apply to the others. Therefore it is very interesting with him, it is really on one level, it is not the doctor speaking with the patient, but it is indeed one level, the whole exchange. Therefore it is very pleasant."

Conventional wisdom holds that with the shift from HIV "exceptionalism" toward "normalization" through treatment, the expert position of the HIV patients is attempted to be undermined and power to be reclaimed by physicians: "It is more than probable that medicine will try to push its virulent claim to power in the field of AIDS at the expense of those groups they so far, like it or not, had to cooperate with due to their own powerlessness" (Dannecker 1997: 17). Impotence is to be shared, power to be kept. While there is, of course, some truth to this argument, I prefer to draw on the approach of Kaufman (1988), who argued that the dichotomy between medical power on the one hand and patient autonomy on the other fails to grasp the assumptions about the boundaries of medical authority (and, I may add, patient autonomy) that are held by patients and practitioners alike.

---

[68] Dannecker described prevention as "the key word of the forces organizing themselves in the shadow of medical impotence" (1997:12).

After reviewing theoretical approaches that discuss the role of the patient and his/her position in the health care system, I will argue firstly that the patient as expert was and is – also in the admittedly exceptional field of HIV/AIDS – to some degree a fiction and that both people with HIV and their physicians remain ambiguous about their mutual relationship. Secondly, I will argue that although medicine gained power back through treatment, this new power of treatment only partially translates into new authority for the physician.

## 3.1. CONSUMING MEDICINE

The "patient-as-expert" is an ideal that partly draws upon and further constructs the ideal of the "patient-as-consumer" as developed since the 1960s. Traditionally, the doctor-patient relationship in Western medicine is described as paternalistic, a view which was vividly expressed by the sociologist Parson (1951), who compared it to the parent-child relationship (Beisecker and Beisecker 1993). The paternalistic position of the physician and the corresponding role of the patient have been challenged since the 1960s. Reeder, who was among the first authors to reflect on the shifting role of the patient becoming a consumer, named as two of the main reasons for the new role definition the "orientation of medical care away from 'treatment' to 'prevention'" and "the growth of consumerism as a social movement" (1972: 407).

According to Reeder, who wrote his article well before the spread of HIV/AIDS, the focus of attention in medical care has shifted toward the prevention of chronic diseases "as the control of acute and/or infectious diseases has been accomplished" (ibid.: 407). Although this task certainly has not been accomplished, different factors did indeed contribute to a shift toward chronic sickness. These factors include firstly the increasing knowledge on how to prevent disease that leads medicine to expand its sphere of competence to the time before an eventual disease may occur. Secondly, the new possibilities to determine probabilities of future diseases help to define populations and risk which therefore become the concern of the medical specialists in the diseases they are at risk for. Thirdly, an expanding market for preventive activities and products is being developed. While according to Reeder curative or emergency care is "the seller's market", in preventive medicine the patient has to be encouraged and persuaded that s/he is in need of medical services, thus introducing elements of a "buyer's market" into health care.

With patients merely "at risk" for disease or having in many cases asymptomatic diseases yet remaining for prolonged and often uncertain treatment in the health care system and being commonly required to undertake profound lifestyle changes, physicians are also increasingly confronted with the rather troublesome social and subjective sides of their patients (Radley 1994)[69]. One response to these developments in the United States was the creation of a new specialty of Family Practice in the 1960s with the ambition of treating "the whole patient" and providing coherent long-term care (Conrad 1987).

Ideally, a consumerist relationship is shaped by different assumptions than a paternalist relationship and it produces different patterns of interaction. In a paternalist relationship, the doctor controls information, access to treatment, and decisions taken while the patient is expected to cooperate and comply. The patient has neither choice nor responsibility while the doctor decides, based on his/her standards of "good medical practice", what is best for the patient. Typically, this type of interaction takes place in a closed system between the – often institutionally independent – doctor and the patient without consultation or intervention of third parties. In contrast, the consumer-patient ultimately chooses the health care provider(s) s/he wants to consult, listens to their opinions, and makes his/her own decisions. This interaction takes place in an open system since the patient may consult several providers while the physician with his/her opinion loses authority and should base his/her work on all the information available, including external sources such as specialized physicians and clinical trials. The autonomy of the patient-consumer is also enhanced by gaining information without having to consult a physician, i.e. through public access to health information. Autonomy and responsibility are shifting from the doctor to the patient[70]. This shift also entails that the patient, like any consumer, should engage in "doctor shopping" until s/he finds the health provider or the com-

---

[69] As Kleinman noted: "Chronic medical patients, as I have repeatedly noted, are thought of as problem patients by their care givers" (1988: 249). These thoughts remain quite unquestioned when Kleinman provides a "method for the care of the chronically ill" (ibid.: 227ff.) through a series of "several practical steps the physician can undertake to get at the patient's model and negotiate with the patient over any conflicts between the lay and biomedical models" (ibid.: 239). Wright and Morgan (1990) provide a rather different perspective on the "problem" patient by focusing on why and by whom patients receive the "problem" label. They find that the organization of clinics around teaching often creates problems for patients, and that "patients may be labeled a 'problem' if they fail to submit to a physician who expects to be the authority" (ibid.: 593). Patients may also violate the rules of "good" behavior in order to assert more control: "Such strategies may be particularly common among patients with chronic diseases, who develop a high level of knowledge about the system and their own condition, which they may use to achieve their goals and to participate more actively in decisions regarding their care." (ibid.: 957).

[70] In a rather nostalgic perspective, Kleinman criticized this consumerist interaction and distinguished it from the "fundamentally moral" interaction found in other societies and earlier times, an interaction lost to the contemporary American physician: "Another example is the passive acceptance by biomedical practitioners of a doctor-patient relationship that is just another instance of consumer-client interactions characteristic of market economy. This economist model represents the diffusion into biomedicine of the most powerful contemporary model of relationships throughout North American society. It runs counter not only to patient-doctor models in other societies' healing traditions but even to the earlier model of a fundamentally moral relationship in medical practice that characterized North American society until several decades ago." (1995: 39)

bination of different providers that best fits his/her needs for a given problem (Beisecker and Beisecker 1993).

With the patient-consumer as a central figure in health care, his/her preferences and attitudes become of central importance to evaluate and structure health care (Huby 1997). While market researchers try to elicit the hidden desires of their customers, researchers in health care – anthropologists amongst them – increasingly focus on the patient's needs and views[71]. This focus on the patient is also reflected in the development of patient-centered medicine that parallels and partly overlaps consumerism in medicine. As described by Silverman and Bloor (1990), who studied patient-centered medicine in different medical settings, modern medical discourses move away from the mere concentration on the body and instead increasingly include the social space between doctors and patients as a therapeutic instrument in its own right. They believed that this movement might reverse the developments, analyzed by Foucault (1996), from a person-oriented medicine to the clinical gaze on the body in the late eighteenth century. Nevertheless, they counter the assumption that integrating the patient's subjectivity into the consultation challenges the asymmetry between doctors and patients. Such an assumption "depends upon a vision of power that censors or silences speech. Yet, as Foucault (1979) showed us, power is at its most effective when it encourages speech" (ibid.: 23). By encouraging their patient to speak about subjective perceptions and by eliciting their explanatory models, doctors may through patient-centered medicine increasingly extend their sphere of competence and influence to include the patient's feelings as well.

## 3.2. SOCIAL SCIENCE AND MEDICINE

The focus of the social sciences on the "illness" aspects that the patient carries into the health care process and on his/her satisfaction with care partly responds to the needs defined by medical professionals to better understand their patients. Studies on "patient satisfaction" (Hall et al. 1988; Hjortdahl and Laerum 1992; Schmittdiel et al. 1997; Winefield et al. 1995), approaches for a patient-centered medicine (Branch et al. 1991; Byrne and Long 1976; Levenstein et al. 1986), or attempts to

---

[71] To quote Paula Treichler who placed the emphasis on the patient in the context of anthropological theories dominant in the 1980s: "Current conventional wisdom is that the patient's view must be honored; the physician is, therefore, urged to understand the patient's cultural construction of reality, to read the native text. This fits nicely into current ethnographic theory. George Marcus and Michael Fischer (1986), for example, argue that *dialogue* is the underlying metaphor for ethnography today. This has a pleasing and contemporary ring to it and seems in one sense perfect: the social in dialogue with the physical, the cultural with the natural. Yet, as Atwood Gaines and Robert Hahn (1985: p. 4) observed, 'for many anthropologists, Biomedicine is *the* reality through the lens of which the rest of the world's cultural versions are seen, compared, and judged'" (1992: 75, emphases in original).

elicit the patient's "explanatory model" of illness (Kleinman 1980) thus also stand in a tradition of making patients more comprehensible to their doctors. Obviously, illness-centered approaches may therefore be criticized for being in the service of medicine as well as for increasing the asymmetry between doctors and patients. As Taussig remarked in his well-known article, "there lurks the danger that the experts will avail themselves of that knowledge only to make the science of human management all the more powerful and coercive. (...) It is a strange 'alliance' in which one party avails itself of the other's private understanding in order to manipulate them all the more successfully" (1980: 12).

In an interview by Charbonney with Swiss physicians working in the field of HIV/AIDS, a Swiss HIV specialist nicely illustrated how physicians readily appropriated the concept of "illness" to assess and describe their patients' views as false consciousness or "prejudice" to be challenged by medicine. Asked about the problems he faced with patient compliance, the physician answered: "This is a very complex question. First of all, there are problems linked to the images people make of their sickness and to the prejudice prevalent about medication. (...). Patients though only reluctantly speak about their ideas. For one reason, they might barely be tenable when confronted with a scientific approach. Some time ago for example I was stunned by the behavior of a patient until I found out through third parties that this patient was absolutely convinced that medication would arouse the rage of the virus, which would take revenge through increased aggressiveness. In this context also an 'eco-toxico-manic' ideology might be mentioned. It consists of rejecting everything artificial and synthetic" (Charbonney 1998: 4-5). Remarkably, the physician did in the example he recounted not even assess his patient's explanatory models in the personal encounter, but relied on information provided by third parties. What he thus found to be the patient's ideas did not seem to support a better understanding between physician and patient, but rather helped to distance the patient's views as exotic and inferior to a scientific approach.

Taussig proposed a shift in perspective from the patient's illness toward the "clinical construction of reality": "The doctors and the 'health care providers' are no less immune to the social construction of reality than the patients they minister, and the reality of concern is as much defined by power and control as by colorful symbols of culture, incense, amulets, fortune-telling, hot-and-cold, and so forth" (1980: 12). Since the early 1980s, the clinical and scientific construction of reality has turned into a major focus of the social sciences, though, according to my impression, with only limited effect on the physicians' and scientists' belief into the objectivity of their knowledge. They, of course, stand on firm ground in their belief. Modern science has become the single most important means to establish matter of fact in the modern Western world (Hagendijk 1990), and medicine serves as the discipline both to represent it paradigmatically to the public and to establish its authority (Lambert and Rose 1996). Researchers in the field of medicine and physicians therefore have the best possible background to claim knowledge and fact and to represent nature "as it is". Working in a clinic and becoming familiar with medical theory and practice, I experienced the strength of this claim myself. Similarly, it has also affected other social scientists entering the field. It is therefore not surprising that the distinction between disease and illness as an attempt to distinguish between scientific knowledge and lay beliefs in the medical encounter have emerged as the first discursive devices of medical sociology and proved to be of lasting success (Atkinson 1995).

As Cassell, a physician, proposed, "let us use the word 'illness' to stand for what the patient feels when he goes to the doctor and 'disease' for what he has on the way home from the doctor's office" (1976b: 48). The magic moment in the doctor's office that causes the transformation from subjective illness to objective disease in Cassell's description is the doctor-patient encounter. It is this encounter where patients' illness "beliefs" and doctors' disease "knowledge" enter into dialogue and frequently clash. The analytical dichotomy between disease and illness helps to organize the clinical encounter by sorting out patients' complaints which do not fit into disease categories as "belief", a more elegant word than terms avoided such as "superstition" (Lock 1988: 3). The distinction thus not only serves as a model to distinguish between biology and culture, professional and lay (Atkinson 1995), but at the same time reproduces these categories by liberating what is seen as objective from anything that does not fit the picture as subjective. As Benoist and Cathebras (1993) noted, the distinction between disease and illness reveals a similar underlying problem as psychosomatic medicine and psycho-immunological or bio-psychosocial approaches: they do not succeed to escape the Cartesian dualism by a holistic concept of the mind/body[72], but they provide subtle returns to the dualism and reify the distinction by creating modified concepts of the interaction between mind and body.

The dichotomy between disease and illness found its most widely used application in medical anthropology through the explanatory model approach developed by Kleinman (1980). Kleinman described the construction of illness experience as the casting of sickness as a "natural" phenomenon into a particular cultural form, a task which is accomplished through the health care system. Kleinman himself put the term "natural" in quotes (ibid.: 72), yet without providing further precision of his definition of nature and the reasons why and how he seemed to distrust it. In his more recent writing, Kleinman (1995) provided a critique of his earlier position, explaining his ambivalence about the explanatory model approach and finding the

---

[72] For critical discussions of the mind/body dualism, see for example: Scheper-Hughes and Lock (1987), DiGiacomo (1992), Lock (1993a), Kleinman (1995), Strathern (1996), Honkasalo and Lindquist (1997).

disease/illness distinction less and less tenable. As Good pointed out in his interpretation of Kleinman's explanatory model approach which he preferred to call "meaning-centered" (a term that he also put it into quotes as he found it dated in retrospective), the approach provided the means to elicit patients' understanding of their sickness as the "native's point of view", yet it also showed that disease belongs to culture, too, and thus is as open for analysis of how it is constructed as illness is (1994: 52, 56)[73].

Ironically, but hardly surprising, illness and disease are in my experience the only analytic and discursive devises that penetrated the medical community from the social sciences[74]. Establishing illness as a perspective worthwhile to be considered by the doctor may therefore also help to reinforce the distinction between the physician's knowledge (derived from the body) and the patient's belief (located in his/her mind). Meanwhile, anthropology and sociology have gone quite a long way in trying to overcome the illness-disease dichotomy with its attribution of knowledge and fact to disease and belief to illness that reaffirms the asymmetry of explanatory power between doctors and patients. Still, it seems quite daring, if not impossible to speak, for a change, of the "doctor's belief" and the "patient's knowledge". The difficulty expresses a deeply rooted understanding that science and medicine express "truth", an understanding which is difficult to be challenged even when keeping the numerous studies of the social and cultural construction of scientific facts in mind. With that difficulty in mind, I have my doubts about the rhetoric of the patient as expert or the patient as consumer.

---

[73] Nevertheless, medical anthropologists and sociologists who base their research on the explanatory model approach tend to focus their analysis on patients and their perspective. This bias may partly be due to the fact that Kleinman as a psychiatrist was in his own words "animated by a clinician's gaze" (1995: 6), which made his approach more appealing to investigate the patient than the doctor. Furthermore, the bias also represents the interests of physicians who quite often are involved in decisions on the allocation of research funds to medical anthropologists and who may prefer to increase their knowledge on patients instead of having their own ideas investigated.

[74] In the already cited interview by Charbonnay with physicians working with HIV/AIDS patients, the interviewer asked whether non-medical disciplines such as psychology, sociology, or anthropology might be helpful in dealing with low adherence to medication. A physician answered: "Psychology surely might. I would be very interested if a psychoanalyst some day would analyze our ideas about health, our readiness to take risks, our feelings of invincibility, and things like that. That might help to resolve some situations where we really try to understand but don't find the key for it. Other disciplines might also help to elucidate these questions, especially in reference to collective or transcultural ideas about sickness and healing" (Charbonney 1998: 9-10). I find this statement less surprising in the physician's ignorance of the fact that these questions have been intensely investigated and elucidated by the sciences mentioned. What troubles me more is the physician's taken for granted assumption that research she does not know about does not exist.

## 3.3. INTERACTING FROM EQUAL TO EQUAL?

People with HIV in our study group described the quality of the doctor-patient interaction as the central aspect in choosing health care, and they highly valued continuity and comprehensiveness of care as a basis for the doctor-patient interaction. The doctor-patient interaction, supported by a continuous care relation, tends to favor the general practitioner over the HIV clinic and seems to account for the increasing popularity of general practitioners with a prolonged time of the infection (Lang et al. 1998)[75]. The emphasis on the doctor-patient interaction as a central factor for patient satisfaction with health care is common in medicine, as various studies show. Hall et al. (1988) for example showed that satisfaction had the most consistent statistical relation with physician behavior, including most importantly the amount of information provided by the physician, and it appeared in their study that patients of higher social class received more information and more communication overall. Hjortdahl and Laerum (1992) found that a personal doctor-patient satisfaction and continuity of the relationship increased chances of the patient being satisfied with the consultation. According to Schmittdiel et al. (1997), patients who could choose their physician were more likely to be satisfied than patients who were assigned a physician. Both continuity of the relationship and the possibility to choose the physician are not given in the HIV center were the physicians tend to change every year.

---

[75] We asked people with HIV to rate their satisfaction with health care in the HIV center and in the general practice and to account for their rating. Satisfaction was greater in the general practice, and the positively valued interaction with the general practitioners was the main reason given for this rating. In contrast, problems with the doctor-patient interaction in the HIV center were most commonly given to account for the lower rating for centers. Other reasons than the quality of the doctor-patient interaction, including for example the medical competence of the physician, were less frequently named to account for (dis)satisfaction both with the general practitioners or the HIV center.

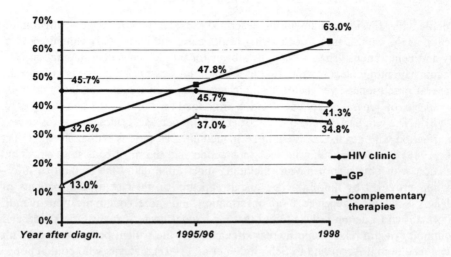

*Figure 6. Changes in health care during the course of the infection*[76]

As figure 6 indicates, HIV care through a general practitioner increased from being used by 32.6% of the study group after their HIV diagnosis to 63% in 1998, thus the percentage of people visiting a general practitioner for their health care approximately doubled from one to two thirds of the group. On a much lower level, the use of complementary therapies[77] initially also increased from 13% of the study group after diagnosis to 37% in 1995/96. After 1995/96, it leveled off to 34.8% in 1998. The use of complementary therapies therefore remained at around one third of the study group which corresponds roughly to the average share of the European population using complementary therapies (Fisher and Ward 1994). In contrast to general practitioners and complementary therapies, HIV care provided by the specialized HIV clinics was consistently used by almost 50% of the study group.

---

[76] Health care in the year after HIV diagnosis was assessed retrospectively in the interview of the 1995/96 study visit for the Long-Term Survivor Study. Health care in 1995/56 was also assessed in the same interview and corresponded to the health care at that time. Health care in 1998 was assessed by questionnaire for the present study.

[77] The number includes therapies undertaken both with and without therapists.

*Table 12. Patterns of health care*

|  | n | Valid % |
|---|---|---|
| GP | 14 | 30.4 |
| HIV center | 7 | 15.2 |
| Complementary therapy | 2 | 4.3 |
| GP + complementary therapy | 6 | 13.0 |
| GP + HIV center | 4 | 8.7 |
| HIV center + complementary therapy | 3 | 6.5 |
| GP + HIV center + complementary therapy | 5 | 10.9 |
| No care/therapy | 5 | 10.9 |
| Total | 46 | 100.0 |

Table 12 focuses on if and how individual persons combined different types of health care at the time of the questionnaire study in 1998. 50% of the study group limited themselves to using only one type of health care: 30.4% attended only a general practitioner, 15.2% an HIV clinic, and two persons (4.3%) exclusively used complementary therapies. 13% of the study group combined health care through the general practitioner with using complementary therapies. 8.7% attended both a general practitioner and an HIV clinic, and 6.5% attended an HIV clinic and used complementary therapies. 10.9% combined all the three types of care/therapy we asked for, and the same percentage did not use any type of health care. To summarize table 12, exclusive care through a general practitioner was the most common type of health care. Fewer people (a total of 19.6% when summing up the people with and without additional complementary therapies) combined a general practitioner with a specialized HIV center. The fact that only two persons did not combine complementary therapies with orthodox health care indicates that in the case of HIV/AIDS, the term "complementary therapies" is indeed more adequate than "alternative therapies" to denominate therapeutic approaches not belonging to orthodox medicine. While exclusively using complementary therapies thus was rare, not using orthodox health care was more common. A total of 15.3% or seven people in our study group (when summing up the 10.9% without care/therapy and the 4.3% with complementary therapy) neither attended a general practitioner nor an HIV center.

As the HIV clinics are organized around educating the assistant physicians which usually remain in the clinic for only one year, patients are confronted with ever-changing physicians. A patient following the regular monitoring visits, which are suggested to take place every six months, sees a physician twice before the next physician takes over. The change of physicians at the HIV centers may at best be somewhat annoying, yet doesn't cause problems in the doctor-patient interaction and in health care, as described below by David Burki, who combined health care for general problems through the general practitioner[78] with HIV monitoring at the clinic and with different complementary therapies. He preferred the clinic for HIV monitoring due to the competence of the physicians and their direct access to laboratory testing. With his personal background as a very self-secure, well-informed and well-educated person, his limited expectations in the interaction, and with his good relations with the senior physician whom he knows on a first name basis, he sets the terms of his encounter with the physician himself:

> "When I have a physician for the first time, then I actually tell him right away what I want. I say, I want my lab, I want this and that. And if we have a little time left, we can talk a bit in general or whatever comes up. That's what I want from him. There is nothing else I want from him. And I do not allow him to do anything I am not convinced of. (...). I actually know what I want, and either he accepts that or else I would simply have to say that I need someone else, but over all these years I really never had to. If things really get difficult, I go to X[79]. (...). The only disadvantage {of the HIV clinic}, but that's a problem for everybody, I know that, is that the physicians keep changing. Sometimes the physician is well prepared when I come, he read at least a few pages in my medical history. But then there are those who start reading when I arrive, and mine for heaven's sake is thick like this[80]. And then they sometimes start thinking what might be due now, and go look for it, and then I have to say: Listen, you don't need to look too far, I have come for this and that. You realize whether they are prepared or not. (...). And I like to come and go quickly. When I make an appointment, I also say exactly how many time intervals I need, I can really say I need exactly this period of time."

It seems difficult to describe the patient-consumer better than the way David Burki did so himself: he "shops" for different aspects of health care amongst different providers, he tells his physician what he wants of him, and if the physician is poorly prepared, he knows what needs to be done according to the protocol of the Swiss HIV Cohort Study in which he is enrolled. If there is some spare time, they might talk a bit, but he feels the talk to be just as important for the physician's well-being as for his own:

> "I usually have a good talk with the doctors, but on the other hand they are also happy if they for a change have a patient like me who has no problems."

Having "no problems" seems to refer both to his physical state with good laboratory values and good overall health as to his social and personal situation. These factors support his consumerist approach to health care. David Burki largely corresponds to what the HIV specialist Luca Granges described as the "American gay

---

[78] Consulting the general practitioner primarily for non-HIV-related problems was also found to be common in a study among women with HIV in England (Madge et al. 1998).

[79] First name of the senior physician.

[80] He indicates about 5 centimeters.

ACT UP[81] type" who in his view represents the type of person most compliant with treatment regimens:

> "The American gay ACT UP type, that's the ideal type, he struggles through everything, he is fully convinced of carrying things through. They are easy and over-enthusiastic. This type is, I wouldn't say a rarity, but far more seldom in Switzerland, it is … a cultural phenomenon."

In describing this type of patient whose "easy and over-enthusiastic" attitude facilitates compliance as "a cultural phenomenon", Luca Granges supports the anthropological view that health care cannot be separated from the social and cultural context in which it takes place. In a study conducted in France and the United States, Feldman created a stereotyped opposition between "France where the patient rarely questions the prescribed treatment and the physician rarely lays out several options for a patient's decision and the United States where the patient is well informed and takes an active role in the treatment, often suggesting or refusing specific therapies in accordance with his or her knowledge and desires" (Feldman 1992: 347). I am not in the position to make cross-cultural comparisons, and I wouldn't deny that differences exist between the two countries and that some of the paternalism of the physician was lost in the last decades. Yet I argue that consumerism only partially applies to most doctor-patient interactions.

Many people with HIV in our study group do not fit the image of the patient-consumer or do not want the type of relationship with their physician as described by David Burki. To Jeff Dijon for example, "trust" was a central aspect of health care since he relied on the interaction with his physician and on the information provided by him. He changed from the HIV clinic to a physician specialized in infectious diseases due to the constant change of physicians at the clinic. Though he described the interaction with the individual physician at the HIV clinic as generally being good, he distrusted the clinic because he believed that important information was lost with the change of physicians:

> "I do not succeed in trusting the center. (…). The relation was very good, very nice, but I prefer to have only one physician. You cannot change all the time. If a physician knows you, it is not necessary to explain the same problems to him every time because he knows you. But if he does not know you, he might miss things. (…). Even if it weren't for AIDS, if I had a serious disease, I would first go to the center to initiate treatment, and then I would go to a private physician. That's how I see it. What is a hospital for? You go there in case of emergency, to react immediately, and then you go elsewhere."

---

[81] ACT UP stands for "AIDS Coalition To Unleash Power". As described by ACT UP Philadelphia, it is a volunteer organization that "stands almost alone in its use of empowerment-based grassroots organizing, aggressive non-violent direct action tactics, and its analysis of the AIDS epidemic as a political crisis that can be solved". " ACT UP still accepts no drug company or government funding" (http://www.critpath.org/actup/ projects.html, August 21, 2000).

In Jeff Dijon's description, the lack of a long-lasting relationship is causally linked to the medical quality of care. He consequently saw the role of the clinic in short-term interventions and initiation of treatment and the role of the private doctor, in his case also a specialist, in providing continuity of care. His ideal doctor would be a family/general practitioner who provides not only continuity of HIV care, but comprehensive care for all health problems, a task not accomplished by his physician specialized in infectious diseases:

> "And I would like to have a family practitioner, as my parents do, a doctor to whom I go all the times for my health. (…). If, for example, I get the flu tomorrow, the flu isn't serious, every doctor can heal it, but my doctor couldn't do it. If I break my leg, a generalist can heal it, but my doctor can't."

The quality of the doctor-patient interaction is not an end in itself, a means to make the patient (or the physician) feel more comfortable. While Jeff Dijon believes that a physician who does not know you will also "miss things" in the consultation, Eliane Dutoit directly relates the quality of the interaction to the possibility of deciding for antiretroviral treatment:

> "He doesn't tell me to do things I don't want to do, he hasn't put me on medication, and he doesn't advise it for me, and that's great. With my way of thinking. I think I would get along with him if medication were required, I think we could work together, as long as they are nice and they treat me with respect."

The importance attributed to the personal relation with the physician indicates a profound ambivalence toward the "new" role of the patient as expert or consumer. On the one hand, all the patients we talked to describe elements attributed to the consumer-patient. In the above examples, Jeff Dijon changed the health care provider until he found a setting where he finds the relation of trust he was looking for, and Eliane Dutoit wants a physician that doesn't decide for her if medication is needed, but instead works together with her. On the other hand, the equality claimed by a consumerist description of the doctor-patient interaction as well as the expertise of patients remained limited in the perception of the people with HIV. Most people do not feel capable of independently evaluating medical knowledge and making their free choices based upon it. Instead, the physician serves as an interface between medical knowledge and the patient, s/he organizes and interprets it and to some degree shapes the decisions taken by the patient through this role. This ambivalence is also summarized by Andrea Meier who switched, as already expressed in her narrative introducing this part, from "information" to "translation" when trying to grasp the role of the physician:

> "As far as I am concerned, a physician doesn't have to tell me what I have to do, he has to inform me. (...) Although, it actually means more than providing information, it also means, somehow, translating medicine to ordinary people."

While there is not only a clear demand, but also a practice of people with HIV to decide on care and cure, there remains uncertainty concerning one's ability to deal with the information provided. As Andrea Meier further reasoned, her uncertainty is based on the very fact that knowledge ultimately remains with the physician who has the techniques to see into her body where he discovers things she can neither see nor notice and would not know about without the clinical gaze. The inside of her body thus becomes territory unknown to herself, yet familiar to her physician:

> "I for myself see nothing, and without all these techniques they have nowadays, the blood tests and all that, I would never get the idea. Actually the whole thing is totally abstract. It happens through my physician; it is through him that I know about it. Physicians are exploring it, always more and more in depth, but a person who is simply living her life does, as in my case, not even notice it. And then I wonder sometimes: Maybe there are people with it who simply don't know it. Who do not know." (Andrea Meier)

The clinical gaze (Foucault 1996) privileges the physician with knowledge inaccessible to the patient, knowledge about the interior of the body. In the case of an asymptomatic HIV infection, it is only through this knowledge, gained through medical explorations into the body, that the infection comes into existence. In fact, people may be infected without knowing about it and thus without being labeled as sick.

In the description of Jeff Dijon, the unknown territory that only the physician has access to, that he is supposed to explore, to elucidate, and to translate to his patient, is extended to include not only inside of his body, but also the world of researchers. These two areas receive in his statement a curiously similar status:

> "He explains everything to me, everything that happens either in my body or amongst researchers, he answers my questions. He takes the time to answer my questions. He gives me details I didn't even ask him for."

Doubts concerning patient expertise are expressed not only by people with HIV, but also by their physicians. The well-informed HIV patient is popular in the discourse of physicians who tend to attribute a positive value to the idea of a symmetrical relationship linked to an interaction between equal partners. Nevertheless, the notion of professional authority returns in their descriptions in more subtle terms:

> "Our patients are very well informed, therefore the interaction can go rather far, because they have read, they went to conferences, to congresses, they have patients associations. There is this category of patients where the interaction is rather exceptional, because you can talk from equal to equal, in a way, although it is clear that ultimately it's us who are holding the information. Certain patients are very demanding, we should always have the latest information, and then they sometimes have expectations that go rather far in terms of comprehending things and in terms of getting explanations, although they do not necessarily grasp everything you tell them. Of course it is our duty to know how far we can go. And then there are the patients who do not understand very much, who do not necessarily want to understand, they are, I would say, not different from other patients. It's quite the same for every disease; there are patients more interested into the disease and then there are others who let themselves be carried a bit more by their physician. (...)."

ck: And for you, the well-informed patients, as you call them, are they easier for you
or do they also create problems?

Both are possible. There are patients who might not handle this load of information. I
really believe it is very variable, it can be very pleasant to discuss with people who are
very up-to-date, and it is clear that you always have to take care how they handle that
information, and if it also doesn't mean too much stress for them to know all that without really being able to handle things because they ultimately lack precise comprehension." (Andreas Bauer)

Although Andreas Bauer described an interaction "from equal to equal, in a
way", ultimately it is the physician who holds the "information" which stands in
opposition to the lack of "precise comprehension" on the patient's side. The physician also has to decide to which degree he can transfer his information to the patient
without assuming too much comprehension and putting the patient under too much
stress, and he has to take care not to be carried away toward too much openness by
the delusion of an equal interaction. Such considerations on the degree of asymmetry and authority necessary and inevitable in the doctor-patient interaction though
tend to be restricted to the case of well-informed patients. Andreas Bauer and other
physicians interviewed tend to dichotomize their HIV patients into the informed and
the uninformed, using as criteria the extent to which patients have access to and
integrate medical knowledge into their understanding of HIV/AIDS, i.e. by reading
articles and attending conferences. With the uninformed patients, asymmetry is
never questioned.

While Andreas Bauer as an HIV specialist argued with "information" and "precise comprehension" in favor of physician authority within the doctor-patient interaction, Markus Mader, a general practitioner who described himself as the advocate
of his patients, argued for the need to limit patient autonomy when it comes to the
patient's choice of physician. He strongly favored patient autonomy and patient
empowerment and tried to integrate them into his medical work by basing the interaction as well as decisions taken on the views and attitudes of the patient[82]. While he
thus stressed patient autonomy within the doctor-patient interaction, he would prefer
to limit it in the structure of the health care system. In his argument, patients
changing physicians undermine with their "shopping" his ideal of the general practitioner as providing coherent long-term care:

"And furthermore we have a system where the patient can opt out of everything, and
we make it very easy for him, and that's another thing to reconsider. Is that helpful? I
am very doubtful about it and I think that the *Hausarztmodell*[83] provides a good

---

[82] See his narrative introducing chapter 5.

[83] The *Hausarztmodell* ("general practitioner model") is a medical insurance model where the general
practitioner serves as case manager and gatekeeper. Usually, the patient initially has to visit his/her
general practitioner who may, if required, refer him/her to a specialist or a hospital and who subsequently coordinates all parties involved. In the case of Switzerland, the patient is limited in his choice to

option. In the case of an HIV patient in the *Hausarztmodell*, he has certain obligations and in return he receives care within a framework where everybody knows his role and function. In the long run that would certainly be much more sensible than patients who go shopping. Something here, something there, and things get confusing and cause expenses."

It seems that each physician is inclined to limit patient autonomy in the field were s/he sees his/her own specific strengths within the field of medicine. The specialist argues with his knowledge to limit patient autonomy in the doctor-patient interaction by emphasizing that he is ultimately the bearer of the "precise comprehension" of medical knowledge that also the well-informed patient does not have access to. The generalist argues against patient autonomy in health care models in order to ensure a coherent long-term care relationship that should in turn facilitate patient autonomy within the doctor-patient interaction. He therefore favors health care models where what he sees as his specific strengths, i.e. providing coherence and continuity of care, become a compulsory element of health care. These models strengthen the general practitioner's position not only toward specialists which Markus Mader defined as his "assistants for special tasks", but also toward patients who lose one aspect of their autonomy, namely changing physicians.

### 3.4. AUTHORITY OUTSOURCED

While combination therapies in the field of HIV/AIDS, as I outlined so far, brought back the power of curing to medicine, they only partially translated into new authority for physicians. The egalitarian doctor-patient interaction, which has been especially stressed in HIV care under therapeutic impotence, remains controversially discussed by patients and physicians alike. The negotiations on the role of the physician and the patient in the consultation cannot be separated from the shifting position both of the individual physician and the doctor-patient interaction within medicine. On the one hand, antiretroviral combination therapies contribute to a shift of competence from the generalist to the specialist. On the other hand, the doctor-patient encounter loses its central position in health care as laboratory results, specialist consultations, or economic and political negotiations gain importance. These developments reflect processes also taking place in other fields of health care.

Authority shifts amongst physicians according to their professional education and institutional location: general practitioners, though having the legal right to prescribe antiretroviral treatment in Switzerland, often feel incapable of managing the complex treatment regimens and refer their patients to a specialist at an HIV

---

general practitioners enlisted by the insurance companies, and s/he has to stay with one general practitioner. Insurance fees are intended to be at least 10% lower than in common medical insurance models (http://www.vhz.ch/open/patienten/vhzpatienten.htm#Hausarztmodell and http://www.medicus.de/quality/html/hausarztmodell2.html, May 24, 2000).

clinic. The new medical power thus may put the general practitioner in the paradoxical situation of having his/her professional authority and autonomy undermined, at least in terms of the curative aspects of medical work. A consequence, which might be generalized to the whole health care system under the influence of increased specialization and health technology, is that the general practitioner redefines his/her profession by emphasizing the interaction with the patient, i.e. the caring aspects of his/her work. Losing authority to the specialists in terms of treatment competence is being compensated by becoming the expert and advocate of the patient, thus by claiming authority over the complementary key discourse to "competence" and curing in medicine, the discourse of "caring" (Good and DelVecchio Good 1993). Taking over the role of the "patient's advocate", translating medicine to the patient, listening to the patient's view and trying to ensure that the patient's view is valued in his/her course through medical institutions corresponds much to what medical anthropology has been asking from the physician. Yet, this definition of the role of the physician is not only responding to new patient demands in "the current period of consumer interest in patient-centered care" (Kleinman 1995), but also to an increased emphasis within medicine on specialized knowledge.

The specialist receives a new scope of action through treatment, giving him[84] a new and often emotionally charged perspective on his work, as described by Luca Granges:

> "I find it very exciting to work with people infected with HIV. It is an enormous challenge, I like to do it, even if it is straining. (...). HIV/AIDS also is an enormous tragedy, although I have the feeling that lately we have been seeing fewer heavy cases. It is also an enormous challenge to be allowed to live in a time and to see that now, for the first time, that things move ahead, that we have something to offer."

Luca Granges expressed excitement and relief as he witnessed and participated in the ongoing transition. While the general practitioners interviewed were supporting the new treatment option as a chance for their patients, they were already during our study more cautious about treating asymptomatic persons, and they never expressed as much enthusiasm for treatment as specialists did. This difference in valuing combination therapies is partly linked to the fact that specialists had been much more confronted with the feeling of powerlessness than generalists. For one reason, HIV/AIDS is the focus of their work and they devote the main part of their professional time to it. For the other reason, they were more confronted with sick and dying patients than generalists, as the outbreak of AIDS is often the reason to refer a patient to the specialist. They therefore were and still are more exposed than most general practitioners to the agony and powerlessness through the confrontation with sick and dying patients and the frustration of not being able to act. Yet the spe-

---

[84] During my several years of working at an HIV center, HIV specialists working as senior physicians at the HIV centers were, as far as I remember, exclusively male.

cialist also has a fundamentally different outlook on treatment than the generalist since he is indeed the one who has to "offer" treatment while a majority of generalists expressed doubts concerning their professional competence to prescribe combination therapies.

Given unequal competence concerning combination therapies, it is not surprising that therapies have a varying effect on the doctor-patient interaction according to the position of the physician in the medical system. A strong statement in favor of relocating authority and control over HIV back to the medical sphere was brought forward by an assistant doctor at an HIV center. He described the moment when treatment enters the doctor-patient interaction as a turning point when the patient is confronted with his/her limited ability to control the infection, and the physician may reclaim this control as the patient becomes uncertain:

> "Almost all HIV positive people with a favorable course say, well, that's because I live healthily, because I don't drink any alcohol, because I can deal well with the sickness, etc.. They say, in a way, I with my will can fight the HIV infection. There are many who say that. And then they say: well, I don't need that, this medication. And somehow I don't find that too bad because during that time they live well. And this illusion, I think, you shouldn't necessarily take away, should you? When the question of treatment arises, then things get difficult for a while, because that's when they get insecure. Although it is a bit mean, for us that is, of course, precisely the convenient moment to say: now, you don't worry, now I take over." (Franz Jann)

With the new power of curing, the aspect of caring loses some of its importance and also some of its problems for HIV specialists. How the emphasis shifted from caring to curing when the "very efficient treatment" became available was described by Claude Keller. When asked if HIV patients pose specific problems to him, Claude Keller recounted how he had established a formal exchange on patient care with a psychiatrist before combination therapies were available, an exchange that did not continue on a formal level at the time of our interview:

> "I found that I had specific problems {with HIV patients}, but that was a time when we did not yet have the very efficient treatment, so I had something like a Balint group with a psychiatrist, and that worked well. But now probably I am also more experienced and I think that I do not have too many problems anymore."

De-emphasizing caring aspects when treatment is available is a common process in medicine. As an anonymous author wondered in a letter in reaction to an article appearing in the *Annals of Internal Medicine* entitled "What Is Empathy and Can It Be Taught?" (Spiro 1992), caring might even interfere with the proper use of treatment: "However, at the risk of sounding sacrilegious, I ask if empathy is really necessary for the highly trained scientific physician of the 1990s? We all know that too much emotional involvement (empathy?) may interfere with making good sound scientific judgments; I raise the question of how empathy enters into our modern sophisticated technological treatment of patients. Is empathy simply a remnant of the days past when the physician did not have the modern tools of treatment?"

(Anonymous 1992: 700). In the case of HIV, the caring aspects are also by specialists not described as obsolete or contradictory to the implementation of treatment.
Instead, they tend to be shifted to the field of compliance/adherence, i.e. to guiding
and supporting the patient in the attempt to follow the requirements of the treatment
regimen[85].

Yet the new power that treatment brings remains partial also for the specialist.
Firstly, not only the means, but also the limits of the physician's authority lie in the
medication itself. The medication takes on a symbolism of power on its own. It is
charged with power that directly works on the body of the person swallowing it and
that is both hoped for and feared by people with HIV. Part of the medical power
thus shifts from the person of the doctor towards the medication s/he prescribes, a
process further described in chapter 4.2..

Secondly, authority is not simply shifted from the generalist to the specialist, but
it partly leaves the domain of the individual physician and the doctor-patient
relationship. Atkinson described the importance attributed by social scientists to the
doctor-patient interaction as an attempt to keep medical work analytically within
comprehensible borders: "Nevertheless, the consultation between patient and
practitioner is but one locus of medical discourse. It does not capture the complex
organization of modern medicine. Indeed, an obsessive focus on the one-to-one
clinical consultation makes the tone of so much medical sociology and anthropology
almost nostalgic for a simpler age of medical work" (Atkinson 1995: 148).
Meanwhile, information is generated and decisions are taken increasingly beyond
the sphere of the practicing physician. Data to base decisions are produced in the
laboratory, treatment decisions are taken through specialist consultations and based
on treatment guidelines derived from clinical research, and health care is influenced
by political and economical institutions. Authority is thus outsourced to and claimed
by third parties, and the physician, especially the general practitioner, may move
closer to the patient, since they share their relative lack of power. Stressing a
symmetrical relationship might be a strategy of the physician to fraternize with the
patient when facing the loss of authority to actors beyond his/her sphere and competence and thus finding him/herself in a structurally inferior position similar to the
one of the patient. In that sense, the feelings of alienation and loss of control when
confronted with medicine commonly attributed to the patient (Kaufman 1988) may
apply to a varying degree also to the physician. In this process, the interface
between general practitioner and specialist as well as between practicing physicians
and medical science may become more controversial, as will be shown in chapters 5
and 6.

---

[85] See chapter 4.5. on compliance/adherence and chapter 5.3. illustrating the specialist's emphasis on
adherence as the "caring" aspect of his work.

Treatment guidelines, which aim at helping physicians base their decisions on evidence from basic and clinical research, play an increasingly important role in the routinization of new technology and treatment. As outlined in chapter 6, this process of guiding the physician's work partly parallels, partly tries to counter an increased influence exerted on medicine by institutions beyond the medical sphere, including patient rights groups, private corporations like insurance companies, and the state. Beisecker and Beisecker found that "medical consumerism can produce its own paradoxes by creating new paternalistic situations whereby patient's rights advocate, insurance company, or the Health Care Financing Administration (...) assume the paternalistic role once held by physician" (1993: 55). This situation though might not be all that paradoxical. The doctor-patient interaction might be liberated from some (though, obviously, not all) of its paternalistic and asymmetrical aspects by the very process of relocating authority beyond the doctor-patient interaction, including – as will be further discussed in the following chapters – to medical technology, medical treatment and its demands for "compliance", to medical science and treatment guidelines, or to social and economic demands from without medicine. In that sense, I believe that as much as the rhetoric of patient autonomy under therapeutic impotence only partially reflected the doctor-patient interaction, moving antiretroviral treatment toward routine treatment only partially translates into a new physician authority in the doctor-patient interaction.

# CHAPTER 4

# HIT EARLY AND HARD?

## JEFF DIJON: ONE DAY THINGS WERE GOOD

When I got my test result, I didn't really change anything at all. In the long run, maybe, I might say that it did change things a bit, I got a bit more isolated, but nothing else. I take care not to transmit it, I watch what I am eating, and that's all. Once I tried meditation, it's not easy to meditate, so I stopped it because my cat would always disturb me. I didn't go for medical monitoring right away. I was infected in 1986, or 1987, I don't exactly remember, and I only started to go to the HIV center shortly before we met, not before. I went there because I was tired, and I didn't feel well, but I don't know if that was psychic or something related to HIV, I have no idea. But I was not happy there, the doctors kept changing. Now I go to Doctor X, I go there quite often, once every two months, every six weeks, every month. He initiated treatment and takes blood, and every time there are differences.

Starting treatment was easy; I practically never forgot it, maybe once or twice. My doctor said that side effects occur mainly with persons that are very weak; they may have many of them. He said that people in my situation, who are doing more or less well, don't have many side effects, practically none. I started with the bitherapy about a year ago. Well, actually it was a triple therapy, but I did not tolerate the third medication well, I had stomachaches. So he gave me a new medication, I don't remember what it was, but I did not dare to take it. Oh, I remember, it was *Crixivan*, and I have 3TC and *Zerit*. With that third medication I took in the beginning, I had many tablets to take; it came up to 19 tablets a day, that's a lot, that's compelling. The two other medications are no problem to me. I take them twice a day, once in the morning, once in the evening. That's not too annoying. It's mechanical, I don't think about why I take them, that's it.

I don't take *Crixivan* because you have to take it an hour before meals, or two hours after, and I wouldn't tolerate that, or I would take it too close before meals. I would not succeed in respecting the hours. Mainly because I take lunch at any time, I have no specific lunchtime. As I don't know when I will eat, I will not take a medication and then tell myself in one hour I will eat, you see, that's annoying. I can't do that, and actually I don't want to do that. And at noon I am not at home, and I would have to take it with me. I don't want to start a treatment when I don't feel capable of carrying it through. And then there are risks with *Crixivan*. Both things annoy me, the regimen and the possible side effects, although it is not sure that I would really get them. When I first started treatment, I only thought that I want to make that cure. Now I get afraid when I read medication directions.

Taking medication in the morning is no problem, I am alone, I am not disturbed. Normally, in the morning, I get up, eat breakfast, go to the bathroom, you see, that's well organized, everything goes well. But the problem is the evening. When I am with friends, or when I am not at home, I don't want to come back to take them. Even when I am at home, I might forget if I am with others, but otherwise, when I am alone, then I think of it.

When I had the stomachaches in the beginning, it didn't really make me think about my disease. But, maybe, more so than I think. Actually, there was a short moment when I was not feeling well. It's true, that was around the time when I started taking these medications. Well, there is also the problem of getting the treatment going, let's say that frightens you. If you feel bad because of your medication, you think of the disease. I don't think of it, I never think of it and I wouldn't want to think of it.

It was tough when my doctor suggested treatment to me, it knocked me down, so to speak, it really frightened me. I don't know how I got used to it, I think you get used to everything. I told myself we would see how it goes. At the moment, it gave me the impression of moving closer to the disease by starting treatment, you see. And then I got used to it. Even when I was a bit weak or depressive – not really depressive, rather depressed – I did not feel ill otherwise. Maybe a little bit psychically diminished, because it is all in your head. The difficult thing with this disease is to remain lucid, calm. You must not give in to panic or think of it all the time. I think that's the problem, to escape from it both with your head as well as with your body.

I had a rather difficult moment when I was told that I should take treatment, I only get a bit aware of it now. My doctor suggested I take antidepressants, and that was good for me. He told me that I can take them for a long time, and when I feel ready we will try to stop them, but I still take them. I don't remember how long I was on treatment without taking them, but not for a long time, maybe a few months. First I didn't feel their effect. Actually I don't think about it anymore. It is like a miracle, suddenly you feel well. I did not realize that one day things were better than the day before, it's not how I felt it. One day things were good, and that was it.

It was during this time, when I had already been taking the antidepressants for a few weeks, that I started taking cocaine again. I think that I did not feel the effect of the medication yet. I had stopped taking drugs a long time ago, in 1989. I started taking cocaine last November, and then for two or three months I took it every day, so I had problems stopping, but I didn't have the money anymore, so I had to stop, I didn't want to steal. So now I make myself a present once a week. It stressed me a bit that I started again, I was disgusted. Well, there are many things that cross your head in that moment, and they always are contradictory, you are content and at the same time disgusted, because that's not something to do, it's not natural and not normal to take that shit, and at the same time it is good. So you are never at ease. You feel guilty, at least I feel guilty. When I take it I curse myself and at the same time I am content and well. It's unbearable.

I don't really know what to except of the medication. As it is a long-term treatment, I don't really expect anything specifically. Well, in the short term, I think I will do what my doctor tells me, I will take my medication for three years, he told me that for three years, at least, I was more or less compelled to take the medication, and beyond that you don't know, we will see in three years. I do what he tells me. My ideal would be to be told: bravo, you won, you don't have the virus anymore, you don't have to take your medication anymore. It would be good if they announced that to me. But as this will certainly never happen, or at least not now, where research is, it is not possible that it will happen, I am pleased for the moment when I am told that my viremia is more or less stable, I don't expect anything more than that.

***

While HIV care and treatment in the general practice long remained of marginal interest and virtually no studies empirically analyzed it (Kidd 1997), general practitioners' care for people with HIV and their prescription of treatment started to receive more attention with the new medical and economic potential of combination therapies. General practitioners in Switzerland are, unlike their colleagues in some other countries, allowed to prescribe antiretroviral treatment. In France and the Netherlands (Redijk et al. 1999) for example, general practitioners are not allowed to initiate treatment, and in Australia (Smith et al. 2000), only general practitioners passing a specific state exam and engaging in ongoing medical education on HIV/AIDS can prescribe antiretroviral medication. In the present chapter, I focus on the prescription of antiretroviral therapies in the general practice and their usage by people with HIV. I try to elucidate some of physicians' and patients' motives against prescribing or using treatment early in the infection, as suggested for example in the prominent editorial by David Ho (1995) who called for early treatment under the martial title "Time to Hit HIV, Early and Hard" (see chapter 2.3.). The attitudes of patients and general practitioners are put into the broader context of a newly changing treatment discourse.

## 4.1. USAGE OF ANTIRETROVIRAL TREATMENT

In the absence of medical treatment, HIV care of asymptomatic patients tended to be characterized by the loss of meaning and content, to be bound to dissolve or to orient itself along episodes of sickness unrelated to HIV, thus illustrating that "a nonprescribing doctor presents a contradiction" (van der Geest et al. 1996: 160). Jonas Ender described the care relation with his patient as having become highly uncertain in its very existence before the discussions of treatment options in 1996 brought new meaning and content:

> "I have known her for many years, and I was the one who had to tell her she was HIV positive. And that was, I think, the only time I had to give someone a positive test result who did not know it anyway. And after that she used to come for general monitoring and CD4 testing. That went on like that for a longer time, I somehow just followed her up and checked if everything was all right and much more than that I somehow could not do. Except maybe, if the cell values had fallen, to give her *Baktrim* or whatever. And, then she did not come for a prolonged period of time. She came, I think, once in 94, that was probably the last time she was with me. I did not even really know then if she would come again. (...). And then she came again around the end of the past year, brought a viral load from your study for the first time, and explicitly asked me: so what's going on now? (...) and I suggested repeating the test since I didn't have any new results, and I got practically the same values. (...). Then we actually discussed the pros and cons of these therapies over several consultations, as far as I could. I also looked for information, mainly through these official statements of the Federal Office of Public Health."

Later in the interview, Jonas Ender reflected on his role as a physician in a situation where there was virtually no action to be taken and no option to suggest:

> "For a while I simply assessed her CD4 cells and somehow I just watched a bit. On the one hand, 'yes, it's still okay', but, well, for a while it was also a situation where I asked myself: Well, what am I actually doing? Is that any good for her now? Is it more of a reassuring or a frightening factor, or whatever?"

The possibility of treatment reduces the doubts concerning one's role as a physician and the fear of becoming mainly a "frightening factor" without having to offer anything in compensation. Even for a physician like Jonas Ender with a rather critical attitude towards treatment, and in a situation when the patient decided against treatment, the sheer possibility of treatment meant that the consultations became more frequent, powerlessness was replaced through possibilities of action, follow-up visits were transformed into intense discussions. Although combination therapies thus re-introduced meaning and content also into the care of asymptomatic patients and bear the potential of bringing the physician his active role back, their usage in the general practice nevertheless remained comparably low, as shown in figure 7.

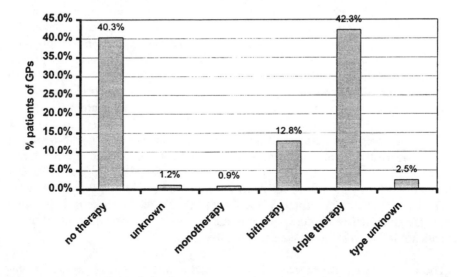

*Figure 7. Antiretroviral treatment in the general practice*

The general practitioners in our study cared, according to their information, for a total of 691 HIV/AIDS patients. 40.3% (n=273) of these patients did not take any type of antiretroviral treatment at the time of our questionnaire study, only 0.9% (n=6) followed a monotherapy, 12.8% (n=87) followed a bitherapy, and 42.3% (n=287) followed a triple therapy. Of 1.2% (n=8) of their patients, general practitioners did not know if they took treatment, and of 2.5% (n=17) they did not know which type of treatment they took. On the whole, between 58.5% and 59.7% of all the patients followed antiretroviral treatment. This number is close to a study conducted amongst HIV/AIDS patients in Dutch general practices in September 1997, thus only a few months before our questionnaire survey. In the Dutch study, 55% of general practitioners' HIV/AIDS patients had already started treatment (Redijk et al. 1998).

When comparing the percentages of antiretroviral treatment amongst HIV/AIDS patients of the general practitioners in our survey to the percentages of treatment in a sample of patients in the Swiss HIV Cohort Study SHCS (Bassetti et al. 1999)[86], one major difference is found. In the SHCS study, the percentage of patients taking triple therapy was with 69.0% clearly higher than amongst the patients of general practitioners. The percentages of patients in the SHCS taking bitherapy (17.5%) and monotherapy (0.7%) were comparable to the ones we assessed in the general practice. On the whole, 87.2% patients in the SHCS took antiretroviral treatment. This difference may be to some extent due to the fact that patients are often referred to the HIV center by their general practitioners when laboratory values worsen and treatment seems indicated. Nevertheless, the study by Bassetti et al. showed that also amongst asymptomatic patients[87] in the Cohort Study, the percentage of triple therapy was with 59.0% clearly higher than amongst the entire population of general practitioners' HIV patients. It can be concluded that general practitioners' HIV/AIDS patients are less likely to take triple therapies and/or general practitioners are less likely to prescribe them than their colleagues working in the HIV centers.

The differences in the usage of antiretroviral treatment according to the care setting are also visible when comparing antiretroviral treatment between general practitioners' patients with or without additional care by an HIV center. Of the 691 patients cared for by our sample of general practitioners, only 46.9% (n=324) were also under care at an HIV center. While 69.4% (n=225) of the patients under additional care at an HIV center took antiretroviral treatment, only 50.4% (n=185) of the patients not followed by an HIV center took treatment.

The comparison between general practitioners and HIV centers reveals institutional differences in the interpretation of clinical trials and guidelines and their transformation into the daily work of the physician which cannot entirely be explained through medical reasons. Similarly, studies throughout Europe also show

---

[86] The data was assessed from September to November 1997, thus only slightly earlier than our questionnaire study taking place in January/February 1998.

[87] Clinical category A according to the 1993 revised CDC classification system (Centers for Disease Control 1992).

geographical differences in the prescription of antiretroviral therapies. A comparison of antiretroviral treatment in specialized HIV centers throughout Europe showed that changing toward a triple or even quadruple therapy occurred earlier in Central Europe (including Switzerland) and Northern Europe than in the South. The authors assumed that "factors other than results of clinical trials affect the use of therapy and might explain the regional differences" (Kirk et al. 1998: 2037). A study that compared the uptake of combination therapies in France and England in 1996 and early 1997 showed that the proportion of patients on combination therapies was greater in France compared to England, especially for asymptomatic patients. The authors give no explanations for these differences which might be for example related to differences in the health care system and insurance coverage. The differences also reproduce a general tendency, described by Payer (1988) as a cultural practice, that physicians in Great Britain generally prescribe fewer drugs and smaller dosages than in France and Germany.

In our group of people with HIV, usage of treatment was clearly lower than amongst general practitioners' HIV/AIDS patients. This might not be surprising since our population of people with HIV was selected in 1995 for having an asymptomatic course of HIV with relatively high CD4 values.

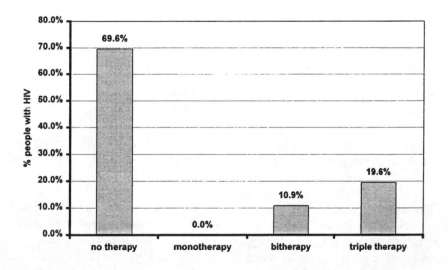

*Figure 8. Antiretroviral treatment amongst people with HIV*

69.6% (n=32) of the group of people with HIV did not take antiretroviral therapies, 19.6% (n=9) took a triple therapy, 10.9% (n=5) a bitherapy, and nobody took a monotherapy. The Swiss HIV treatment guidelines[88] in use at the time of our study stated: "The indication for treatment is given in principle when an HIV infection is documented". The guidelines though named a number of options that might restrict this indication, amongst them the option to delay treatment when a patient has CD4 values above 500/mm$^3$ and a viral load below 5000 copies/ml (SKK/EKAF 1997). Based on this option, we assumed that it was mainly the people with favorable laboratory values as indicated in the guidelines who did not take antiretroviral treatment and that laboratory values were therefore associated to the treatment decision.

*Table 13. Association between laboratory values and antiretroviral treatment amongst people with HIV*

|  |  | Laboratory values | | | | Total | |
|  |  | CD4≥500 and viremia<5000 | | CD4<500 and/or viremia≥5000 | | | |
|  |  | n | % | n | % | n | % |
|---|---|---|---|---|---|---|---|
| Usage of AT[89] | Yes |  |  | 14 | 30.4 | 14 | 30.4 |
|  | No | 11 | 23.9 | 21 | 45.7 | 32 | 69.6 |
| Total |  | 11 | 23.9 | 35 | 76.1 | 46 | 100.0 |

p=0.012

To calculate the association in table 13, we used the laboratory values as measured in 1995/96 for the Long-Term Survivor Study. Since all of the study participants had at that time not taken antiretroviral therapy, these values reflect the situation before treatment, i.e. the basis to decide on treatment. In contrast, the self-reported laboratory values we asked for in the 1998 questionnaire are not only less accurate, but they above all reflect, in the case of patients with treatment, already a treatment effect. They therefore do not represent the laboratory values which were used by people with HIV and their doctors to decide on treatment. The study group was split up in two groups according to the laboratory values indicated in the guidelines.

The usage of antiretroviral treatment was indeed significantly associated to the laboratory values (p=0.012). This finding stands in contrast to the Dutch study on HIV in the general practice already cited above where there was no association found between treatment decision and CD4 values (Redijk et al. 1998). Remarkable in the association between laboratory values and treatment is the re-interpretation of the threshold values given in the guidelines. While the guidelines recommended

---

[88] The Swiss HIV treatment guidelines are elaborated by a national expert group of HIV specialists and published in the bulletin of the Federal Office of Public Health. They are not enforced by any legal or economic measures.

[89] The abbreviation "AT" used in tables and figures stands for "antiretroviral treatment".

treatment for all patients yet gave the option to delay treatment if a person had more favorable values than the threshold values, people with HIV seemed to interpret these values as the first indication to start considering treatment. In our study group, none of the persons (n=11) with CD4>500 cells/μl and viral load <5000 copies/ml took treatment. Amongst the remaining 35 persons with laboratory values below this threshold, still only a minority of 14 persons took treatment while 21 persons remained without treatment. For people with HIV, treatment therefore seemed to be indicated less through their HIV infection, as suggested by the guidelines, but rather through laboratory values announcing that a possible progression towards AIDS might come closer.

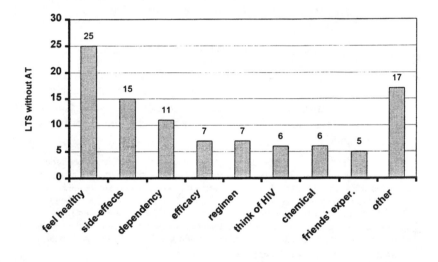

*Figure 9. Reasons against taking antiretroviral treatment amongst people with HIV*

People with HIV not taking antiretroviral treatment were asked about the reasons for their decision (Figure 9). 25 of the 32 persons answering the question said that they did not take treatment because they felt healthy. The incompatibility of asymptomacy and taking treatment was frequently expressed in our interviews. David Burki for example wondered: "why should I pre-treat something when I feel healthy?", and Peter Carreira commented on his decision against treatment despite his CD4-cells having dropped below 500 as follows:

> "{The general practitioner} described the options to me. My attitude is, and that might
> be wrong, and I can maintain it as long as I have no symptoms, my attitude is that as
> long as I am doing well, I do not need treatment. I know that might be against common
> sense at the moment, but it is my subjective feeling, and that's all right with him {the
> general practitioner}. I take a tablet a day for my blood pressure, and that's enough for
> the moment."

The idea of taking antiretroviral treatment is connected to sickness, even for Peter Carreira who easily combined this view with taking preventive treatment against high blood pressure.

The second reason given against treatment was the fear of side effects named by 15 persons[90]. Eleven persons said that they feared dependency from the medication, a factor that is, along with the fear of medication as "chemicals" or foreign agents entering the body, further discussed in chapter 4.2. Each group of seven persons doubted the efficacy of antiretroviral treatment respectively found the treatment regimen to be too complicated, each group of six persons didn't want to think of HIV when taking medication respectively didn't want to take "chemicals", and five persons decided against treatment due to bad experiences of friends.

## 4.2. THE PROMISE OF POWER

For people with HIV, treatment has a very physical quality. Medication is absorbed by the body, it acts within the body, it affects and alters it. Moritz Pedrini who did not take antiretroviral treatment for example contrasted the power of orthodox medication with homeopathic medication he used and which he described as being "barely traces of matter":

> "The difference is that all the medication I inject is homeopathic medication. *Iscador* as well, these are traces, barely traces of matter, and even the basic matter are plants, of organic origin, mainly (...). But the drugs from orthodox medicine are incredibly strong preparations and they are measured in high doses, as far as I know, and then I simply don't know what other effects they have. Besides, I also fear that when I feel supported by such powerful matter, it might somehow weaken my vitality and my will to live; that I would not have to fight myself, but could simply rely on medication that will do it all right for me. That's not so nice, is it."[91]

---

[90] An Australian study amongst mainly gay men found the fear of side effects to be their main reason against antiretroviral treatment (Gold et al. 2000), and in the qualitative part of a Swiss study with patients taking antiretroviral treatment, side effects also appeared as one of the three main types of difficulties with treatment (Meystre-Agustoni et al. 2000). Patients' fear of side effects is also amongst the main reasons why physicians did not prescribe treatment to patients with, according to the guidelines at that time, a clear medical indication for it: in the study by Bassetti et al. (1999) conducted in Swiss HIV centers, patients' refusal against treatment due to fear of side effects was one of the two reasons most frequently indicated by physicians to explain why they did not prescribe treatment to patients with a clear indication for it. The other reason was the physicians' belief that the patient would not comply with treatment (see chapter 4.5.).

[91] The difference that Moritz Pedrini constructed between orthodox medication as a strong force measured in high doses and homeopathic medication which is barely matter at all is not as absolute as he presents it here. As he outlined later in the interview, *Iscador* represented to him a drug that crosses the boundary between homeopathic and orthodox medication, and he therefore also hoped to become independent of it: "Well, it is at the limit, well, *Iscador* in my imagination is, acts like a medication. I am a

Moritz Pedrini believed that, besides having the potential for unpredictable side effects, the drugs as "powerful matter" inside his body would actually weaken his vitality by making his personal fight against HIV unnecessary. The responsibility taken for the infection and the strategies built up to cohabit with the virus and to control its action within the body are questioned through treatment and may even be weakened and become obsolete as they are replaced by the effect of the medication. For the example of antibiotics, Jana Seifert described a very similar antagonism between the processes of her body and the processes induced through medication which are swallowed "from the outside":

> "I simply have the feeling that antibiotics stop something inside of me, and it is something synthetic, it is something, yes, something very aggressive, that I swallow from the outside, that interrupts a process inside of me, an important one, I think. The whole production of antibodies afterwards, that's just a good thing the body does, and I just interrupt the process."

As described in chapter 1, HIV transgresses the boundaries of the body and requires efforts to re-create integrity, autonomy, and control in the face of the potentially uncontrollable virus within. The medication may receive a similar status as the virus itself, entering the body as an unknown and uncontrollable "powerful" and "aggressive" factor from the outside, acting within the body and altering its workings in unpredictable ways. The body, already polluted from the outside through HIV, is now threatened with pollution again, this time through medication.

While Moritz Pedrini and Jana Seifert describe an antagonism between the activity of the body and of the medication, between inside and outside, self and other, Andrea Meier fears that introducing medicine as an external, "chemical" actor into the body might even blur her very ability to make such distinctions:

> "In this uncertainty I simply wouldn't want to take so many chemical things. Maybe then everything really runs out of control, you never know. Now I know why I feel like this, why I feel good or bad, but if I take all that medication, one doesn't know, I don't know anymore, cannot distinguish anymore what I am causing and what the medication is causing, and then I would feel bad anyhow, and that scares me. (...). I already feel scared when I need to have an operation, and I get an anesthetic, and also otherwise, alcohol or drugs or something like that, and my conscience and awareness slip away, and that is somehow scary to me."

In the description of Andrea Meier, treatment interferes with her perception of her body and her self, it makes it impossible for her to distinguish "what I am causing and what the medication is causing" and therefore questions her identity in ways similar to what she believes psychoactive drugs would do. Forces acting inside of her body, yet beyond her control, undermine her coherent and conscious self. Treatment thus introduces a new dimension into the identity of a person with HIV,

---

bit dependent on it, although I could imagine that when I am free of all my duties, I might also be able to do without it."

built up through long, complex, and often difficult processes. It symbolizes a power (Benoist 1989/1990) that may threaten personal integrity and autonomy. Martin pointed out in the case of *Prozac* that the medication is "not an animate being like a therapist, exactly, but neither is it an inanimate object like a stone. Once a person has taken Prozac, it is alive in them; simultaneously, the person has ingested a technological device. Together they form a cyborg, part human, part machine" (1996b: 105). In a speech at the 1998 World AIDS Conference, Jairo Pedraza described how the body under medication might turn into a strange and unknown object. As he found the shape of his body altered through side effects of antiretroviral treatment known as "Crixi belly" or "buffalo hump" (Dong et al. 1998; Viciana et al. 1998), he wondered: "Oh my God, is this my body?"[92]

The image of medication as the opposite of the body/self and its power is expressed through the attributes for medication used by people with HIV. Medication was described as "chemical" and "synthetic", and as "aggressive" and "powerful matter" which alters, weakens or even suppresses processes of the body/self[93]. Artificiality and power entering the body from without are central attributes of orthodox medication which seem to be shared also by other patients. In a study among patients of British general practices, Britten cited a patient describing medication as "an alien force" (1994: 466). Britten interpreted the common concerns about "unnatural" medicines of patients in her study as having a double meaning. On the one hand, medicines are perceived as not naturally grown, just as Moritz Pedrini opposed orthodox medication to homeopathic medication which is "of organic origin". On the other hand, they are not natural to the body: also in Britten's study, patients feared that medicines weakened their body's own power by damaging the immune system or preventing it from working, just as Moritz Pedrini feared that antiretroviral medication might weaken his vitality and Jana Seifert believed that antibiotics interrupted processes inside of her. The ambiguity of evaluating the power of treatment may also follow a cultural logic of medicines. In their review of the anthropology of pharmaceuticals, van der Geest et al. link anthropological perspectives on magic, fetishism, or animism to the more recent research on pharmaceuticals as social and cultural phenomena[94]. They point out that the ambiguous

---

[92] Speech held at the Community Symposium 3, "Facing a future: long-term survival with HIV", June 29, 1998

[93] The arguments resemble the second most important reason against treatment (following the fear of side effects) given by mainly gay Australian people with HIV: "These antiviral drugs are very strong poisons. The last thing I need is to add strong poisons to my body" (Gold et al. 2000: 365). More than half of the study participants agreed with this statement.

[94] "The cultural (symbolic) logic of medicines was discerned by early anthropologists in so-called primitive societies. They called it magic, fetishism, or animism: the belief in the immanence of forces that people attempt to possess, control, and manipulate to their own advantage. Until recently, however, few anthropologists extended that cultural perspective to pharmaceuticals – the synthesized, manufactured,

meaning of power has always been inherent in medicines: "By definition medicines are substances that have capacity to change the condition of a living organism – for better or, in the case of sorcery medicines, for worse" (1996: 154).

The power attributed to medication has its striking counterpart in the presentation of medication by its producers. In the case of the new antiretroviral drugs, the protease inhibitors which led to the highly increased efficacy of combination therapies, power was a common metaphor to describe their efficacy. Two different pharmaceutical companies for example, *Agouron Pharmaceuticals, Inc.* and *Roche Laboratories Inc.*, advertised their protease inhibitors with the metaphor of power. *Agouron* described Nelfinavir (brand name *Viracept*) as "Powerful and easy to live with", a slogan visualized through the opposition of a wild bear showing its teeth and a friendly teddy bear (Figure 10). *Agouron* thus created the ambiguous image of medication as a wild, yet tamed and domesticated animal exercising its power within the body without hurting or destroying it. The advertisement text explains the ambiguous imagery by underlining the power of the medication in fighting HIV, while refuting two common fears about medication, namely the difficult treatment regimen and the possible side effects. According to *Agouron*, the power of the medication reduces the viremia and increases the CD4 cell count while it is characterized by an easy regimen and good tolerance, though qualifying that "people treated with VIRACEPT may experience some side effects" (ibid.: 8).

---

and commercially distributed therapeutic substances that constitute the hard core of biomedicine" (van der Geest et al. 1996: 154).

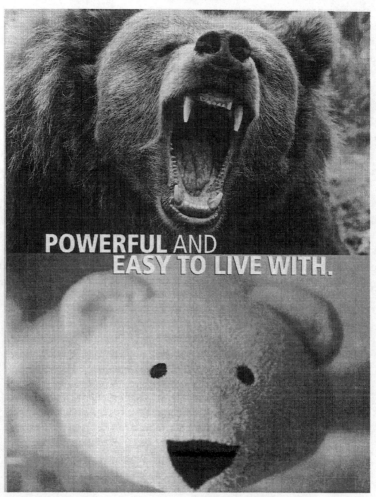

*Figure 10. Powerful and easy to live with*
*Part of an advertisement for* Viracept *by* Agouron Pharmaceuticals, Inc., *published in:* a&u
America's AIDS Magazine, *Vol. 7, Issue 45, no. 7, July 1998, p. 8-10.*
*Copyright © 1998;* Agouron Pharmaceuticals, Inc.; *reproduced here by kind permission of*
Agouron Pharmaceuticals, Inc..

More than *Agouron* even, *Roche* relied on the imagery and metaphors of power
when introducing *Fortovase* as an "improved formulation" of their earlier protease
inhibitor *Invirase,* which was known to be poorly absorbed by the body. Both
*Invirase* and *Fortovase* are based on the substance *Saquinavir*. While *Saquinavir* is
presented as "The promise of power", visualized by a female javelin thrower
attempting to throw her javelin (Figure 11), *Fortovase* is "The power released", the

javelin thrower releasing her javelin. While the images visualize power through the metaphor of athletics, the advertisement text uses a war metaphor which is more traditional to medicine[95]: It states that "FORTOVASE therapy releases more HIV-fighting medicine into the blood compared to INVIRASE®" (p. 115).

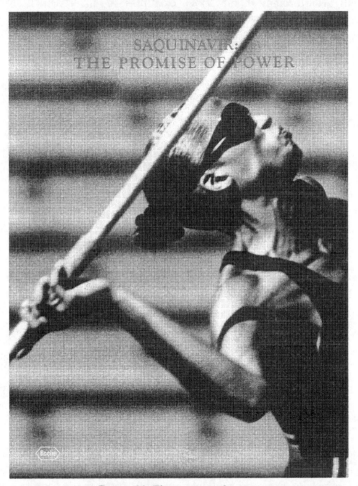

*Figure 11. The promise of power*
*Part of an advertisement for* Fortovase *by* Roche Laboratories Inc., *published in:* POZ Magazine, *Issue 37, July 1998, p. 113-117.*
*Copyright © 1998;* Roche Laboratories Inc.; *reproduced here by kind permission of* Roche Laboratories Inc..

---

[95] See chapter 2.3. on war metaphors.

Pharmaceutical companies presenting their products as sources of power join a long healing tradition. When they advertise their drugs as powerful, they also represent their own power, just as the power of magic reflects the power of the magician and vice versa. The power attributed to the product and the power of its producers are mutually reinforcing. In the above examples of advertisement for protease inhibitors, the power of the pharmaceutical companies producing them is already represented simply by the size of their advertisements, namely three to five pages. Rouse (1992) counted that a quarter of the journal *Science* is devoted to advertisements. He remarked that this fact alone suggests the economic significance of scientific work and that the amount of advertisement in medical journals leaves room for doubt whether it is really the scientific articles that are the meaningful content of these journals.

Pharmaceutical companies increasingly cross and blur the boundaries between the commercial and scientific domain of medicine. As Rabinow has pointed out for the United States, scientists increasingly represent the interests of pharmaceutical companies. The Patent and Trademark Amendment Act that passed US Congress in 1980 and that was intended "to prompt efforts to develop a uniform patent policy that would encourage cooperative relationships between university and industry, and ultimately take government-sponsored inventions off the shelf and into the marketplace" (1992: 172) facilitated this shift. In consequence, according to Rabinow the 1980s saw an increased movement across the university-industry boundary. This movement was supported by economic ties such as sponsorship for research and personal ties as scientists became formally integrated into the biotechnology industry. Companies also took on the symbols of universities by incorporating libraries, organizing conferences and seminars, and hiring scholars to mimic the features of a university.

The increasing affiliation between research institutes and pharmaceutical companies may also be symbolized by the fact that starting in 1993, the journal *Nature* published "a series of bimonthly advertisement-linked features" (Anonymous 1993: 757), thus combining the editorial with the commercial sector of their journals. The first feature was described as "a survey of the ways in which pharmaceutical companies in the United States, Japan and Europe now support research and researchers from academic laboratories. The funds available from these sources seem to be growing rapidly, and are increasingly regarded by biomedical researchers as valuable supplements of the funds available from public grant-making agencies" (ibid.: 757).

The power of the pharmaceutical industry, which is omnipresent in the entire field of medicine, is also enacted in medical conferences. The visual and social center of the World AIDS Conferences for example is the commercial sector where pharmaceutical companies present themselves and their products. Their booths are remarkable for their height and size, and they attract more public through their gifts and gadgets than many scientific sessions do. Having attended several medical conferences, I keep my computer mouse on a pad advertising *"Norvasc®"* and *"Zoloft®"* (whose use I do not know) and my notepad in a briefcase from *Pfizer* (whose activities I only learned of since they sell *Viagra*), and I drink my breakfast coffee from a *New England Journal of Medicine* mug. Although I do not have the professional capacity to prescribe drugs, *Merck Sharp & Dome* paid my room in a luxurious hotel when I was attending the World AIDS Conference in Geneva. When I look up the official definitions of HIV and AIDS or the list of currently available antiretroviral drugs, I use the *Sanford Guide to HIV/AIDS Therapy* provided by *Antimicrobal Therapy, Inc.*. Aware of the fact that a therapy guide published by the producers of drugs might create unease, the publishers reassure me in the first page: "You, the user, should know that the SANFORD GUIDES are not prepared for any single pharmaceutical company or distributor. Though it is distributed by multiple companies in the health care field, the SANFORD GUIDES have been independently prepared and published since their inception in 1969. The SANFORD GUIDES are not subject to any form of approval prior to publication. Decisions regarding content are solely those of the editors" (Sande et al. 1998).

Despite this reassurance, pharmaceutical companies reach their goal in establishing themselves as an important source of information on disease and treatment for the physician. In our interviews, an HIV specialist described the relations with the pharmaceutical industry, along with conferences, journals, and the Internet, as one of the main sources of information for his department. When asked how he and his department gained knowledge on treatment, he answered:

> "I must say that for the moment I have so many other things going that I cannot primarily inform myself. We have interns who are on the Net. Well, we have connections to the industry. X who is presently in charge of the HIV center sits in the committees that write these guidelines. I read what is being published, although that is all a year out of date. (...) I was in Vancouver last year, and I will certainly go to Geneva next year, and now this year I go to Toronto, and then for the next few months I will again know the latest things coming out. We have people on these mailing lists, every morning they load their fifty things down from the Internet. Well, I simply don't have this time." (Luca Granges)

With the rising cost of health care, the influence of the pharmaceutical industry on health care providers became a publicly discussed and controversial issue, as may be illustrated by an advertisement by a Swiss health magazine (Figure 12). The advertisement shows a physician – male, senior, authoritarian, adorned with the paradigmatic technical devises of his profession – who states: "We physicians are not paid by the pharmaceutical industry". The subtitle of the advertisement contradicts him: "*PULStip – the Swiss Health Magazine. Who reads it, knows better.*"

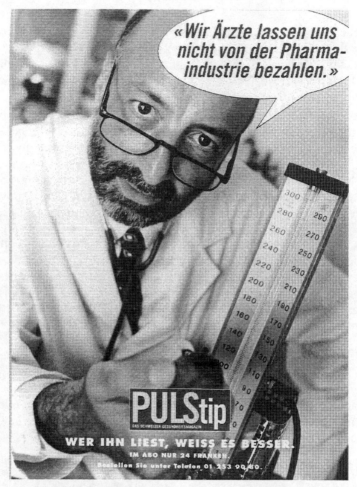

*Figure 12. We physicians are not paid by the pharmaceutical industry*
*Advertisement for* PULStip – the Swiss Health Magazine. *In:* K-Tip, *Issue 12, June 14, 2000,*
*p. 34.*
*Copyright © 2000;* PULStipp; *reproduced here by kind permission of* PULStipp.

## 4.3. NEGOTIATING TREATMENT

When interviewing general practitioners, I was astonished by their doubts concerning the use and efficacy of antiretroviral treatment for asymptomatic patients[96]. My astonishment may have been intensified as I came from the setting of specialized HIV care where doctors were more enthusiastic about antiretroviral treatment. François Neher for example, a general practitioner who is well-experienced in the care of HIV/AIDS patients, described his doubts about antiretroviral treatment as so fundamental that he felt relieved when a patient did not want treatment:

"I think great progress has been achieved in the quantitative sense, but qualitatively? Can we as orthodox physicians really oppose something to this disease that heals it? The answer is still a clear no. Despite the newest studies and the disappearance of the viral load, this virus is everything but eliminated. It is simply less frequently found in the places where you look for it. And as long as it is like this I do not feel obliged to say to a patient: actually you should... In the contrary, I am actually glad when somebody tells me with conviction: listen, that stuff from orthodox medicine interests me no more than marginally. In that case, I feel relieved."

Despite this strong statement of doubt against antiretroviral treatment, François Neher tried to abstract to some degree from his attitudes by adapting his recommendations to his patients. He described how he supported patients when he found them to be desperate for treatment by suppressing his doubts and instead stressing the advantages of treatment:

"I do not have to rub the patient's nose in the shortcomings of this therapy. If he asks me, I can honestly inform him, but if somebody says: listen, I am so desperate and I now urgently need whatever orthodox medicine has to offer, and orthodox medicine certainly has a lot to offer, then I don't say no. I rather say: I do my best and whatever I can do, and I stress the positive aspects and say: crucial improvements of these treatment options have been observed during the last years and what seemed totally uncertain five years ago now seems to be much more grounded. Something like that."

François Neher's patient did not decide to start treatment despite his CD4-cells having dropped below 500. He described how he expected his general practitioner not to put pressure on him to start treatment. He thus confirmed his general practitioner's approach of guiding the treatment discussion through the patient's view:

"As far as AIDS is concerned, I get, so to speak, only psychological care from my general practitioner. The way he deals with it, with his tactfulness and a certain distance, leaving me freedom, that's right for me, I don't have any problems with that. I would have a problem if he had told me, for example after the results I got from the study: Less than 500 {CD4}, now you have to take at least one of these drugs, probably two. I would have had problems with that because I was personally not ready. But it was no

---

[96] In the questionnaires, we asked general practitioners to rate the overall efficacy of antiretroviral treatment on a five-point scale from 'very efficacious' to 'not efficacious'. 14.0% of the general practitioners rated them as 'very efficacious', 54.1% as 'rather efficacious', 28.0% as 'moderately efficacious', 3.1% as 'little efficacious' and 0.8% as 'not efficacious'.

question for him, he said: I suppose you do not want therapy – well, he didn't say it
that sarcastic. And I said: Yes, I think so. And that was it." (Peter Carreira)

Despite physicians' efforts to base decision-making on their patients attitudes
and preferences, their own attitudes remain present in the consultation. Both Gregor
Pfister, a general practitioner, and Franz Jann, an intern in a specialized HIV center,
described the influence of physicians' attitudes toward treatment on their discussion
of treatment with their patients. Gregor Pfister described how he used to discuss
AZT (brand name *Retrovir*) treatment only reluctantly with his patients due to his
doubts concerning efficacy and how he still did not suggest treatment to patients
when he doubted their ability to comply:

"For example concerning *Retrovir*-prophylaxis, at the time when only that was possible, I must say I was not euphoric. I actually haven't seen and read much good about it,
well, I was very skeptical and in that sense, I haven't recommended it to the patients. If
people wanted to take it, I sent them to X. I collaborate also with {the HIV center}, but
I didn't really push them. And now with these new, these triple combinations, which of
course show much better results... I tell that to patients when they come, and when I
feel that they could take it for example concerning compliance."

In the description of Gregor Pfister, the improvement of treatment options
diminished to some degree his reluctance against discussing treatment with patients.
Nevertheless, he still selected the patients he discussed treatment with according to
their assumed ability to comply[97]. In contrast, Franz Jann reflected on how the initial
euphoria over the new treatment options was already being replaced by disillusionment and doubts in regard to the long-term perspective of treating asymptomatic
patients:

"If I may add something concerning triple therapies: In the beginning, we said that the
virus falls to zero, we were all euphoric and thought: okay, now we have the drug, and
we can win over HIV. And therefore we of course tried to push everybody to take
treatment. In the meantime I became less sure of what we were doing to people over
time. I do believe that there is an alleviation for a couple of years, but whether it really
makes a change in the long run we do not know."

When I asked Franz Jann if his disillusionment had changed his treatment discussions with patients, he replied:

"Let's put it that way: when today somebody thinks about starting treatment, and he
just has a slightly elevated RNA, then I might be a bit less convincing, that's possible, I
am more easily satisfied when he says that he does not want it."

The changing attitudes of physicians affect their discussions of treatment with
patients in two ways: firstly, as shown by Gregor Pfister, the attitude toward treatment influences the probability of discussing the subject with patients. Secondly, as
described by Franz Jann, the attitude also affects the manner in which treatment is

---

[97] See also chapter 4.5. on physicians' assumptions about patient compliance.

discussed with patients. According to Franz Jann, as he "became less sure", he might have become "a bit less convincing" in his presentation of treatment to patients.

The sensitivity of patients for the attitudes implicitly or explicitly expressed by their physicians and their influence on the treatment decision became apparent in our interviews with people with HIV. Andrea Meier for example who decided after an intense evaluation to delay treatment described how her physician communicated his attitude to her:

> "He {the general practitioner} tended toward still waiting a bit, because as he said, people were different, and he has known me for a long time, since the infection, and there were people who wanted to try out everything as quickly as possible, and others who trust more – I don't know how to put it – trust more in life." (Andrea Meier)

The influence that physicians exert on the attitudes and decision-making of their patients though is not a one-way process. Rather, patients may influence their physician's attitude as well. The well-informed patient that provides the physician with information and thus may actually guide the doctor-patient interaction corresponds to a stereotype of the HIV-patient and has been described by some of the general practitioners. In addition, patients may also influence their physician's attitudes by the way they are dealing with their infection and by the decisions they are taking. Jonas Ender for example described how he was impressed by his patient's reactions in the face of HIV:

> "And then I have to say she is a stable person, she has something incredibly healthy. And she started saying: What I can do is to live healthily. And she did sports, and now she thinks of starting a new education. I never had the impression that she suppressed anything, but rather an attitude like: I go on living now, and I don't know how long that will last, and I don't limit myself too much, and I can't go for it with an apocalyptic mood. Well, I must say, I am indeed a bit impressed."

Markus Mader is putting the mediation between patient's and physician's attitudes in simple terms when saying:

> "I have the impression that in the end as a physician you have the people that fit you, and you lose the people that dislike that style, they don't come back."

Care and treatment decisions are not straightforward applications of the results of clinical results and guidelines, but include complex social processes. The fact that negotiations between physicians and patients are amongst these social processes is, as shown in tables 14 and 15, explicitly acknowledged and desired both by people with HIV and general practitioners.

*Table 14. Who should decide on treatment? (people with HIV)*

|  | n | % |
|---|---|---|
| Doctor | 7 | 15.2 |
| Patient | 12 | 26.1 |
| Both | 27 | 58.7 |
| Total | 46 | 100.0 |

A majority of the people with HIV in our study group wanted their attitudes to be considered by their physician and wanted to participate in the treatment decision. As table 14 shows, only seven persons (15.2%) believed that the physician alone should decide on the necessity to start treatment, 12 persons (26.1%) wanted to decide by themselves, and the remaining 27 persons (58.7%) believed that the treatment should be negotiated between the patient and the physician.

*Table 15. Who should decide on treatment? (general practitioners)*

|  | n | % |
|---|---|---|
| Doctor | 110 | 20.8 |
| Patient | 21 | 4.0 |
| Both | 399 | 75.3 |
| Total | 530 | 100 |

As table 15 indicates, people with HIV and general practitioners differ in their attitude concerning the treatment decision mainly in one regard: clearly less general practitioners (4.0%) than people with HIV thought that the patient alone should decide on treatment, while more of them (75.3%) believed that treatment should be negotiated between patients and physicians. The percentage of general practitioners (20.8%) thinking that it is the doctor who should alone decide if treatment is necessary was similar as amongst people with HIV.

A majority both of general practitioners and people with HIV thus believed that treatment decisions should be negotiated between patient and doctor. As table 16 though indicates, not all general practitioners suggested treatment to their HIV/AIDS patients and thus offered them the opportunity to negotiate treatment decisions.

*Table 16. General practitioners' reasons against prescribing antiretroviral treatment*

|  | n | % |
|---|---|---|
| Patient rejected AT | 52 | 47.3 |
| Patient has not yet decided | 34 | 30.9 |
| Not suggested | 33 | 30.0 |
| Patient stopped AT | 21 | 19.1 |
| Total | 110 | 100.0 |

Given that the guidelines in principle suggested treatment to all HIV/AIDS patients, we asked general practitioners having patients not taking treatment about the reasons against prescribing it. Patients' rejection of treatment was the reason indicated most frequently (47.3%). Reasoning with patients' preferences in prescribing treatment is consistent with a whole body of research on prescribing behavior in the general practice which showed that physicians link their prescribing behavior to patients' preferences[98]. Remarkably, all of these studies exclusively investigated overprescribing, thus reflecting an underlying or often directly addressed public health concern with costs of medication. In contrast, in relation to the guidelines at that time and to prescriptions at the HIV centers, antiretroviral treatment in the general practice tended to be underprescribed. The common explanation for overprescribing given by physicians in the above cited studies was their patients' expectations for prescription as well as the "the desire to prevent problems in the doctor-patient relationship" (Veldhuis et al. 1998: 27). Some of the newer studies also asked patients about their expectations on prescribing and showed that the physician's perception of patients' expectations did not always correspond to the patient's expectations. Physicians explaining overprescription with patients' preferences might therefore base their decisions on an inaccurate assessment of patients' preferences. These studies found that although patients brought expectations into the consultation regarding medication, the physicians' opinions about their expectations were the strongest determinants of prescribing (Britten and Okoumunne 1997; Cockburn and Pit 1997). Britten concluded from this finding that "patients cannot take all the blame for overprescribing" (1995a: 1084). In the case of general practitioners' prescription of antiretroviral treatment, only a detailed comparison would show to what extent patients' preferences indeed correspond to physicians' perceptions of these preferences.

30.9% of the general practitioners said that they had patients who had not yet decided on treatment. This relatively high percentage reflects that treatment decisions are a process that takes time and intensive negotiations between doctors and

---

[98] See for example: Schwartz et al. (1989), Bradley (1992), Veldhuis (1994), Webb and Lloyd (1994), Britten and Okoumunne (1997), Cockburn and Pit (1997), Veldhuis et al. (1998).

patients. Andreas Bauer described the treatment decision as a process that may take months and may even require the repetition of laboratory tests for the main purpose of proving disease progress to the patient in order to underline the importance of treatment:

> "That's never something done in one consultation. I think it's evident that when I see her the next time, well, then we will discuss it, and then I will suggest to see her again maybe not in six months, but in six weeks in order to discuss it once more, and then little by little she gets used to the idea of entering a period where treatment might be justified. What we often do is reconfirm the results a second time, that means we repeat the tests after three months, they show that the virus is indeed higher than before, and that this is an element that forces us to initiate treatment. You also have to give arguments in favor of starting treatment, and the patient has to develop his ideas and has to be convinced as well, has to look for recommendations, see other people, patients, in order to get other opinions."

While patients' rejection against treatment and patients' indecision indicate that treatment has indeed been discussed in the consultation, 30.0% of the general practitioners that had HIV patients without antiretroviral treatment said that they did not suggest treatment to their patients. It can be assumed that in these cases the general practitioners therefore decided by themselves, without discussing the decision with their patients, that treatment was not indicated. 19.1% of the general practitioners had patients not taking treatment because they had already stopped their antiretroviral therapy. Although this reason was the least frequent, it indicates that less than two years after the introduction of combination therapies, a portion of HIV/AIDS patients could or would not comply with the required long-term continuity of treatment.

*Table 17. Why did general practitioners not suggest antiretroviral treatment to their patients?*

|  | n | % |
|---|---|---|
| Medical reasons | 24 | 75.0 |
| Patient's attitude | 15 | 46.9 |
| Personal attitude | 3 | 9.4 |
| Other | 2 | 6.3 |
| Total | 32 | 100.0 |

The 33 general practitioners that according to table 16 did not suggest treatment to their patients were asked why they did not do so (table 17). Most physicians (n=24) indicated medical reasons against suggesting treatment, i.e. favorable laboratory values[99] or medical contraindications. Given that the guidelines stated that

---

[99] CD4>500/μl and viral load <5000 copies/ml. These values were chosen in accordance with the Swiss guidelines at that time which gave them as threshold values for the possibility of delaying treatment (see also above concerning the guidelines).

CD4 values "play an increasingly subordinate role" for the treatment decision, and that CD4>500/μl and viral load <5'000 copies/ml only meant that one "can for the moment wait with treatment while the further course is being monitored" (SKK/EKAF 1997: 20), it would seem that these physicians could have discussed a treatment delay with their patients instead of making the decision by themselves. While only three physicians gave their personal attitude towards treatment as a reason for not discussing it, 15 physicians had not suggested treatment because they assumed that the patient would not want it. In these cases, patients therefore were not offered treatment because their physicians implicitly assumed, without asking them, that they did not want it. Whether these implicit assumptions are always correct may, in the light of the studies on physicians' prescription habits cited above, be questioned.

## 4.4. SHARING UNCERTAINTY

Medical uncertainty concerning the indication of treatment and lack of knowledge on long-term efficacy offered the opportunity to physicians as well as people with HIV to base decisions on their personal experience and attitude. While scientific and clinical uncertainty concerning treatment may complicate the work of the individual physician, it may at the same time also become a resource to liberate him from the influence of basic and clinical science by increasing freedom in decision-making.

While some physicians react to this open situation by leaving it to their own judgment whether treatment is indicated for their patients, others stress the negotiation between doctor and patient by putting it at the center of the decision-making process. Medical uncertainty thus can support what many general practitioners see as their role and strength in the health care system, namely advocating the patient's view within the health care system. Such an understanding of the physician's role is further strengthened and, as shown in the following chapter, became officially supported in the case of antiretroviral combination therapies since responsibility taken over by the patient is a prerequisite for sustaining a complicated and demanding long-term treatment. As Silverman and Bloor (1990) found in their study, patient-centered medicine is valued mainly when the patient is required to take an important part of the control over treatment to allow its success. Jonas Ender nicely summarized the link between medical uncertainty, complicated treatment regimen, and an emphasis on patients' preferences:

> "For the moment, I am still somehow... well, I can put it that way: I am still skeptical to the point that I have to say that I actually don't know, either. (...) She once came and said that she was confused and everybody was saying something different, and I told her to listen to her inner voice. I mean, so far she came once or twice a year to the physician, and that was it. And then {with treatment} she would have blood taken, and laboratory tests, and medication she has to swallow, and side effects she might get. She has to know why she takes that upon her."

Jonas Ender described his personal uncertainty and skepticism concerning treatment and the fact that treatment requires a lot of energy and time from the patient and may cause side effects. He linked this argumentation to the recommendation he gave to his patient to "listen to her inner voice". François Neher, whose attitudes toward antiretroviral therapies and recommendations given to patients resembled the ones described by Jonas Ender, contrasted his discussions with patients concerning antiretroviral treatment with the discussions of anti-hypertensives:

> "I doubt that science has progressed far enough to make it more or less a compulsory exercise of orthodox medicine to squeeze anybody into the view of HIV held by an orthodox medical practitioner. I do not have the type of arguments as when I counsel someone and say: listen, lowering blood pressure is a good strategy to avoid later heart attacks and strokes. I do not believe that you can say: we physicians understand what HIV is, and that's why you just have to make so and so many blood tests, and below so and so many CD4 cells you have to start treatment, double or triple combination. I believe that all that is not yet a routine of orthodox medicine where you would very strongly have to urge the patient to do it."

According to François Neher, antiretroviral treatment was, at least when applied to asymptomatic patients, still in the experimental phase. Defining treatment as experimental and medical knowledge as provisional let him emphasize the priority of patient decision and control in discussing treatment, similarly as Jonas Ender did. In contrast to antiretroviral therapies, anti-hypertensives received in François Neher's description the position of a proven and doubtlessly useful treatment. He thus constructed an opposition between the two therapies as an experimental versus a routine treatment which are characterized and distinguished by the position and power of patients and physicians in the decision-making process. In the case of the experimental therapy, patient autonomy compensates for the uncertainty in medical knowledge while in the case of a routine therapy, physician authority represents medical knowledge.

In his opposition of experimental and routine treatment, François Neher integrates one of the major elements that Koenig (1988) found to characterize the process of routinization when new procedures move from a status of experiment to the standard of care. Koenig argued that the technological imperative, i.e. the fact that the mere existence of a dramatic new medical device provides a mandate for its continued use, is sustained by social forces. These social forces include the creation of new routines and new rituals, and the transformation of the technological imperative into a moral imperative to provide treatment once it has begun to feel routine. The moral imperative, expressed through a moral tone, derives from a sense of certainty experienced by the physician. François Neher exemplifies the moral tone in his argumentation for anti-hypertensives. It is resisted in favor of patient autonomy in the case of antiretroviral therapies which are "not yet a routine of orthodox medicine where you would very strongly have to urge the patient to do it". Under the condition of medical uncertainty, the patient is given a voice to take over decisions that the physician feels insecure about and responsibility is gladly shared with the patient.

## 4.5. TREATING THE COMPLIANT PATIENT

Physicians tend to stress their patients' attitudes as well as their assumed motivation for treatment and ability to comply with it as central factors in the treatment decision. This position has to some degree been encouraged and supported by the Swiss treatment guidelines. The two patient-related factors that the physician should, according to the treatment guidelines, include into treatment considerations are the patient's motivation for treatment and the expected compliance with treatment. In the version which was in use during our study, the guidelines suggested delaying treatment when "there are indications for insufficient compliance" (SKK/EKAF 1997: 20). In the version updated in December 1999, the insight that "doctors cannot predict who will comply with prescriptions and who will not" entered the guidelines[100]. Nevertheless, the short version of these guidelines still named, as the first two of three factors that should guide treatment decisions, the patient's motivation and expected treatment adherence: "all patients who are 1. motivated for antiretroviral therapy and 2. will be able to take drugs several times a day in the correct sequence and 3. show signs of immune deficiency (CD4 <350/µl or viral load >5'000-30'000 copies/ml plasma) should be treated with a triple combination."[101]

Haynes defined compliance as "the extent to which the patient's behavior (in terms of taking medications, following diets, or executing other life-style changes) coincides with medical or health advice" (1979: 2). Treatment compliance as a field of research that had been growing over the previous decades only became a focus of HIV research with the introduction of combination therapies. The growing concern with compliance in HIV research reproduces the increasing attention the subject has generally been receiving in medicine: Trostle (1988) showed a dramatic increase in research interest between 1960 and 1985: while up to 1960 only 22 articles in English were listed in a cumulative bibliography on the topic, 3200 articles were listed in the *Index Medicus*[102] for the time span of only six years from 1979 to 1985.

---

[100] In the United States guidelines, the same implicit insight lead to the following recommendation: "In regard to adherence, no patient should automatically be excluded from consideration for antiretroviral therapy simply because he or she exhibits a behavior or other characteristic judged by some to lend itself to non-compliance." (Feinberg 1998: 48)

[101] The recommendation is cited from http://www.hivnet.ch/e/index-frame.html, updated December 21, 1999.

[102] The "Index Medicus" contains articles of more than 3'000 medical journals published worldwide. The articles are collected and indexed by the United States "National Library of Medicine" (http://www.nlm.nih.gov/).

One of the shortcomings of compliance research – which is reproduced in its application to HIV treatment – is the limited understanding it gives of factors determining non-compliance. Chesney for example, a leading researcher in HIV treatment compliance, found in several studies "simply forgetting" to be a main reason for non-compliance without further looking behind this quite superficial category (Chesney and Hecht 1998). Approaches that look at non-compliance from the patient's point of view, as Stimson (1974) suggested already in the 1970s, remain rare and barely found their way into mainstream compliance research in HIV. Through such approaches, non-compliance has been interpreted for example as attempts for self-regulation and to assert control over one's sickness (Conrad 1985; Hayes-Batistuta 1976), or it has been shown how the physician's orders compete with other factors in patients' decision-making on treatment (Donovan and Blake 1992).

Trostle (1988) tried to explain such analytical weakness with the narrow perspective of compliance research on patient behavior, a perspective which is determined by a medical view of the patient and his/her relationship to medicines. The contemporary concern for compliance is according to Trostle linked to the growing monopoly of the medical profession over the past century. Compliance researchers therefore mistakenly tend to equate health care dominated by the physician with health management in general. Yet the consumption of medicines is not limited to the rather narrow temporal and spatial boundaries that delimit the dominance of the medical profession: "Labeling patients 'non-compliant' because they follow their own ideas about their own care misses the point that this is what people have done since medicines were first used" (ibid.: 1301).

As research on HIV treatment compliance boomed, the term "compliance" gradually became viewed with suspicion and replaced with "adherence" as its correct counterpart. As a comparison of abstracts on the subject published at the 1996 International Conference on AIDS in Vancouver and the 1998 World AIDS Conference in Geneva shows, the research volume dramatically grew within only two years while the term adherence gained popularity. At the 1996 conference, 98 abstract contained the word "compliance" and 28 the word "adherence". In 1998, 276 abstracts spoke of compliance and 266 of adherence. The comparison shows that the research volume grew by about 400% and, while "compliance" was far more common than "adherence" in 1996, both terms were used about equally often in 1998. An increasing interest of pharmaceutical industries in HIV compliance/adherence paralleled and partly created the growing body of work on the subject. The companies producing antiretroviral drugs now support research and provide tools to enhance compliance as one of their marketing strategies (Maskovsky 1998). They thus follow an established strategy to "increase the visibility of their products and to enhance the company's positive image among physicians and the lay public" (Trostle 1988: 1299).

The change in terminology from compliance to adherence intends to symbolize that the patient is not seen as an obsequious, passive object of medical interventions anymore, but rather becomes the physician's active partner in treatment. As Harley et al. (1998) and Maskowsky (1998) argue, this new image of the patient stands for broader attempts to shift responsibility for health, sickness, and treatment from the health care system to the individual patient. "In fact, adherence plays a crucial role in the definition of the HIV-positive person as the ideal image of the post welfare state consumer: the person that governs itself through adherence" (Maskovsky 1998: 15). According to these authors, the broad emphasis on patients' adherence does not only neglect the economic role of the state and the health care system in providing patients with treatment, it also hides deficiencies of the drugs themselves concerning efficacy and manageability.

Following Foucault, the emphasis on the patient's active and self-responsible role expressed in the term "adherence" as opposed to his/her passive role of following orders through "compliance" may also provide yet another example of the increasing sophistication of power. According to Foucault's historical analysis of power (Foucault 1999, Gordon, 1980 #937), the net of external top-down power is too loose to control everything and everyone; it therefore is complemented by an individualized and atomized power of the individual over him/herself, i.e. through self-control and discipline. Likewise, as medical control of patients' compliance proves to be impossible, the patient is asked and educated to assume control over his/her behavior in order to act self-responsibly according to the physician's prescriptions.

While little conclusive insight into patient compliance/adherence has been gained through research, the one finding which seems to be rather clear is that doctors' assessment of their patients' compliance is inaccurate, or, as Sackett et al. put it, "is no better than flipping a coin" (Sackett et al. 1991: 261). In our interviews, many physicians implicitly or explicitly overestimated both treatment motivation as well as compliance with regular medical follow-up visits and treatment regimens amongst their middle-class patients. Meanwhile, they were doubtful concerning motivation and compliance amongst their lower-class patients, mainly intravenous drug users. André Favre for example described that his well-educated patient who lived a stable upper middle-class life was actively seeking follow-up visits and that he never had to be afraid the care relation might break off. Yet when looking into the medical history of his patient, he realized that he hadn't seen him for more than nine months, although the laboratory values in the last visits had crossed the threshold where treatment was suggested by the guidelines:

"He deals very intensively and, as I believe, on the whole in a good and positive way with his sickness, and he makes his appointments himself. There are so many {patients} you have to remind, otherwise it fizzles out, and in his case you know it keeps going. (...). He is always active. In that sense, no problem, you don't have to worry that anything fizzles out.

ck: (...). He said that the last time you met, his blood values had dropped below the threshold of treatment recommendation at that time, and then the question of treatment was relevant?

Yes, well, since then I simply haven't heard anything anymore, that's a pity. I don't know the current situation anymore. I just still have the...[103] well, that's July 96, and then we monitored again in August 96, the viral load, it was still slightly below these 30'000. And the helper cells had for the first time dropped below these 500. That's the situation I still have. It's simply outdated. Well, I don't know what's happening now." (André Favre)

His patient was aware that he did not return for the follow-up visit although, as he said, his physician had suggested that he should come back three to four months after the last visit[104]. He clearly knew why he did not call to schedule a visit and further blood tests:

ck: "Did you talk with him about the fact that you did not have further blood tests taken?

No, not talked at all. He said, any time in three, four months you come again. And I simply had the feeling that there is no need for it, it is not urgent, I will deal with it by myself. And that is very important to me, that I am actually independent and get along by myself.

ck: And did you for yourself reflect why you did not return to your physician?

Yes. Clearly because I am less under pressure. I like to see him and I always look forward to it. But the contact with orthodox medicine is something that always touches a bit the sphere of paternalism. I expect that I will have to be supported by it again. But as long as it is not necessary, I am very happy to keep a certain independence here, too." (Moritz Pedrini)

While André Favre was confident that he didn't have to worry about continuity of care and only became aware of his patient's non-compliance with suggested follow-up meetings during the course of our interview, Moritz Pedrini was not only well-aware of his non-compliance, but also knew his motives for it. As Moritz Pedrini's narrative introducing chapter 1 shows, he described his life as having been guided too strongly by external pressure. As a consequence of this insight, he increasingly tried to limit external pressure in favor of self-control. Orthodox medicine represented to him to some degree the paternalism characterizing the oppressive society he was struggling against. Antiretroviral medication stood to some

---

[103] He looks up the medical history of his patients.

[104] It was not common amongst general practitioners to automatically invite their patients to a planned or regular follow-up visit: Of the general practitioners with HIV patients in our sample, only 22.5% (n=48) used a system to invite their patients.

degree in opposition to an independent approach to his infection. For these reasons, he wanted to delay this option as long as he felt it to be reasonable. It was therefore exactly the active and self-responsible approach toward HIV which his physician believed to guarantee compliance with medical care that actually caused him to delay care and treatment.

While André Favre overestimated compliance in the case of his upper middle-class patient, Claude Keller, a physician specialized in HIV, generalized the boundaries between compliance and non-compliance amongst his HIV patients:

> ck: "Could you characterize the patients that have more problems either with deciding to take treatment or with compliance?
>
> They are mainly the people who are drug users, or former drug users. They have a relation to the product that is completely different.
>
> ck: Different in what sense?
>
> In the sense that it has an outstanding importance, the medication or the drug has in any case an outstanding importance in their lives, whether it does good or bad. They have a relation to the medication that is completely particular. It's a minority of my patients. On the other hand, for the patients I have here in my practice who are hetero-sexual or homosexual, it is part of their lives. They brush their teeth in the morning, they take their medication, they brush their teeth in the evening, they take their medication. If they get too much diarrhea and it keeps them from working they call me and we change it[105]. It is much more banal.
>
> ck: Couldn't one also imagine that drug use, or this particular relation, might also help to get used to the dependence from the medication?
>
> There is more dependence, but I am not sure if that helps so much. My impression is that whatever doesn't work in life is transferred to the interaction between the sick person and the medication."

To Claude Keller, the boundary that separates compliant and non-compliant patients runs along the lines of HIV risk groups, with drug users or former drug users as problem patients and homo- and heterosexually infected persons as compliant patients. In a pilot study conducted in the United States, physicians in general made a treatment decision based on expected patient compliance even before the first meeting with the patient. The primary source for their decision was the medical history; drug use or mental disorders were seen as interfering with compliance (Erger et al. 2000). A French study found a priori judgments of patient compliance to be a common criterion among physicians when selecting patients for inclusion in clinical drug trials. Intravenous drug users were therefore less likely to be included

---

[105] Claude Keller describes his middle-class patients as tolerating symptoms to the point when they keep them from working. Once their ability to work is questioned by the symptoms, they come to the doctor. This is consistent with a pattern that Zola (1973) found amongst Anglo-Saxon patients and that he generally believed to characterize middle-class and more highly educated patients: the perceived interference of symptoms with work is amongst the main non-physiological factors that triggers the decision to seek medical care. He interpreted this pattern to be rooted in Protestant ethic.

into these trials (Munzenberger et al. 1997). Constructing treatment motivation and compliance along the lines of risk group and ultimately of social class might follow the same logic that DiGiacomo (1999) described for physicians' judgment of the validity of patient reports in research interviews: physicians extended greater credence to those patients who most resembled themselves in terms of social class. The social distance between physician and patient thus shaped their perception of patients' credibility.

It might not be surprising that matching compliance with social class and risk group oversimplifies the problem. Sackett et al. showed that "compliance with long-term medications runs at about 50%, regardless of whether the intent is to prevent or alleviate symptoms" (1991: 251). The popular idea that affiliation to a social group predicts compliance is not supported by research (Maskovsky 1998). It thus seems improbable that compliance with the unusually complicated regimen of antiretroviral combination therapies is as easy for homo- and heterosexual patients as Claude Keller described it. On the other hand, compliance amongst (former) drug users seems to be better than he and many of his colleagues think. Samuels (1990) referred to the widespread "shadowy images associated with intravenous drug use" when provocatively titling a comment with: "Can IVDUs[106] Comply with Conventional HIV Care?". Drawing upon his study in a New York inner-city HIV clinic where he found no differences between drug users and other patients (Samuels et al. 1990), he concluded that they can comply just as much as other patients. Similarly, a study in Geneva found that injecting drug users may delay treatment, but "once they have started it, their compliance is no worse than the compliance of patients from other risk groups" (Broers et al. 1994: 1121). Despite such findings, one of the mechanisms that reinforce the physician's image of drug users as non-compliant was described by Feldman who found in field research amongst HIV specialists that drug users which did not fit the widespread image of being "frustrating, time-consuming, disinterested, and noncompliant" (1995: 138) were not labeled as drug users[107], thus allowing to perpetuate the stereotype by applying it only to people that fit it.

Despite research indicating that compliance with long-term treatment tends to be difficult for all patients and is not limited to any specific group, there are indications

---

[106] "IVDUs" is an abbreviation commonly used in medical talk for "intravenous drug users".

[107] Feldman described the example of a discussion about drug users in a French clinic: "Two residents and two nurses were sharing horror stories about particular IVDU patients, each demonstrating the difficult, disruptive nature of these patients. One resident brought up the name of a patient not previously mentioned. A nurse responded that this patient was not like the others at all and was immediately characterized as cooperative, never coming to the clinic high, keeping all her appointments. Though I had encountered this patient previously, no one had ever identified her as a drug user. Thus, though she used intravenous drugs, this patient was not marked in discourse because she did not fit the definition of an IVDU patient in terms of the meanings constructed by the Rousseau staff" (1995: 139).

that doctors' judgment of patients' motivation and compliance may translate into more reluctance to treat (former) drug users and patients from lower social classes. The study by Bassetti et al. (1999) conducted in the Swiss HIV Cohort Study showed that the main reason for not prescribing combination therapies to patients with a clear medical indication was the physician's belief that the patient would not comply with treatment. The patient-related factors associated with not receiving treatment despite medical indication for it were lower education, current intravenous drug use outside a program, and infection through intravenous drug use. This association between patients' social class and quality of care reflects a common phenomenon in medicine: a meta-analysis summarizing the results of 41 studies containing information on provider behavior in medical encounters showed that patients of higher social class received not only more information and communication, but also higher quality care. These results were consistent with physicians' self-reports of more interest and less frustration when treating patients of higher social class (Hall et al. 1988). Both these studies thus indicate that physicians' attitudes and beliefs about patients' motivation and compliance, which are biased in favor of patients from higher social classes, translate into better care for these patients. Given the biased perception of patient compliance, treatment recommendations that encourage physicians to include expected compliance into treatment decisions might therefore unwillingly support uneven access to treatment[108]. Physicians' beliefs that drug users will not follow treatment might therefore indeed turn out to be correct, but for somewhat different reasons than implied. Drug users may simply be less likely than other patients to be offered treatment by their physicians.

## 4.6. ANTICIPATING THE NEW REALISM

HIV combination therapies were during our study – and to some degree still are – experimental treatments, especially when applied to asymptomatic persons. The introduction of a new therapy does not only create high levels of excitement, but also upsets the routines of clinical practice, causing disorder that cannot be tolerated for long. The desire for routinization of new therapies goes hand in hand with the aims of pharmaceutical companies who want to establish their new products. Koenig (1988) pointed to the irony that the very process which is considered central to evaluate new therapies rigorously and scientifically, i.e. the randomized controlled clinical trial, contributes to the routinization of a treatment in the hospital setting while it is still experimental. At the HIV outpatient department where I worked, new

---

[108] Such an effect may actually be the opposite of what guidelines are intending: including the patient's motivation and ability to comply into treatment guidelines may be inspired by an attempt to empower patients in treatment decisions, thus representing the shift from a more paternalistic towards a more consumerist approach to the doctor-patient interaction and health care, as described in chapter 3. It seems though that only the more powerful amongst patients can take advantage of such attempts for empowerment.

drugs entered the office shelves through clinical trials, to be given out to the study participants. Once the trial was finished, patients could often stay on the drugs without having to pay for them until they were officially approved by the state and thus reimbursed by health insurance companies. Through this practice, new drugs are established and used even before official approval, and the clinical trial, which prolongs the time for a drug to get on the market, is at the same time also a central element in establishing it on the market before it officially enters it.

The time it takes for a drug to be officially approved by the state ("drug lag") is a factor prolonging the time it takes a drug to become profitable. The drug lag has been dramatically reduced for antiretroviral medication, thus accelerating the process of routinization. In the United States, the requirements for drug approval through the Food and Drug Administration FDA were stiffened in 1962 (Bodenheimer 1985) to the point that it may take years for a new drug to be approved. Through a joint effort, people with HIV/AIDS and the pharmaceutical industry have dramatically reduced the drug lag for HIV medication. While people with HIV are motivated by the need to have access to the new therapies before it is too late, pharmaceutical companies enhance their profits by reducing the time until they are allowed to sell their new products. Antiretroviral medication set new records in approval time: "In approving ritonavir, the FDA hit what was then an all-time speed record: just 72 days after Abbott filed its application. So goes FDA approval of AIDS drugs; the trials tend to be stopped the instant that survival benefit is observed – even if that benefit is counted in weeks or months – and the drug is rapidly unleashed upon HIV-positive people by busy doctors who rely solely on the government to determine prescription options. (...). Merck's indinavir (brand name: Crixivan) was the third protease inhibitor to gain approval, an event that occurred only days after the FDA approved ritonavir. Indinavir was approved in just 42 days, breaking the record set by ritonavir" (Johnson 1997: 58)[109]. Fast drug approval not only means economic benefits for the pharmaceutical companies, but it also becomes a symbol for the power of the drug. Without commenting on the symbolism of the approval time or denominating the drug mentioned, which seems to be *Crixivan*, Schulz cited a patient describing the new drug combination prescribed by his physician: "There is another substance, something absolutely new has been added. They have approved it in America within 42 days" (1998: 139).

Obviously, HIV medication set new records in the official process of crossing the continuum from experiment to standard therapy. These records were set in and enabled by the atmosphere of euphoria that characterized the early days of combination therapies. In medical practice, the process of standardization is more pronounced and supported in specialized HIV centers than in private practices. In the

---

[109] Copyright © 1997; Hillary Johnson; reproduced here by kind permission of the author.

former, new drugs arrive earlier through trials and exposure to new developments in HIV research is greater as physicians attend more conferences, read more specialized journals, are visited more frequently by pharmaceutical representatives and sponsored more generously by their companies. In talking with general practitioners, I realized that their position within medicine and their greater institutional, local, and social distance towards basic and clinical research gave them a different outlook on medical knowledge. Health care and treatment decisions are also a product of the physician's position within the medical setting. Unlike HIV specialists, most general practitioners do not attend HIV conferences and do not participate in clinical trials. They are therefore less involved in the production of medical knowledge and profit to a lesser degree from the symbolic and economic capital of these. These differences result in a different application of medical knowledge in practice. The structural and social differences between clinics and private practices may contribute to the higher percentages of patients treated with antiretroviral therapies at the HIV centers as compared to general practitioners' patients. According to François Neher, general practitioners do not widely participate in the first experimental phase of a new treatment which is mainly enforced at the specialized clinics. Instead, new treatment only enters the general practice on a broad scale once it has proven efficacious:

> "The very latest is not necessarily the very best. There is this effect which is quite good, that the university clinic first separates the wheat from the chaff, and that we as general practitioners rather use whatever passed this first filter."

Compared to the treatment guidelines at the time of our study, which in turn reflected the treatment enthusiasm expressed by exponents of HIV research, general practitioners tended to underprescribe antiretroviral treatment. The more skeptical voices amongst researchers started to gain weight around the time of our study. As described in chapter 2.3., by 1998 also researchers and specialists had to some degree sobered off their enthusiasm about treating all HIV patients as early as possible. The initial "euphoria" was gradually replaced by the "new realism", as Peter Piot, director of UNAIDS[110], described the shift occurring between the 1996 International Conference on AIDS in Vancouver and the 1998 World AIDS Conference in Geneva: "If I had to characterize the last AIDS conference in Vancouver in one word, then it would be 'euphoria'. In this conference, it was 'new realism'. Yes, the therapies are efficacious, but there are some 'buts'. The side effects, the resistance that some people develop, and then the young people that were very present at this conference. This is the face of the new epidemic. AIDS will still be with us for a long time" (Lüthi 1998: 68)[111]. The new realism was translated into more cautious

---

[110] The Joint United Nations Programme on HIV/AIDS. See on the Internet under http://www.unaids.org/.
[111] Copyright © 1998; *Neue Zürcher Zeitung*; reproduced here by kind permission of *Neue Zürcher Zeitung*.

treatment guidelines. The United States guidelines of 1998 state: "Although there is theoretical benefit to treating patients who have CD4+ cells >500 cells/mm$^3$, no long-term clinical benefit of treatment has yet been demonstrated" (Feinberg 1998: 47). Factors named against early treatment in the guidelines include the potential for adverse side effects on the quality of life, the potential risk of developing drug resistance, the potential for limiting future treatment options, the potential of transmitting virus which is resistant to drugs, the unknown durability of treatment effect and the unknown long-term toxicity of some drugs. Based upon these risks and uncertainties, rather than proposing a desired course of action, the guidelines summarized current practices as either aggressive or cautious approaches and suggested that either approach should be based upon the patient's decision following discussion with the health care provider.

The Swiss guidelines reflect the growing skepticism towards treating asymptomatic patients by gradually expanding the boundaries where treatment "can be delayed". The guidelines that were in use during our study stated: "The indication for treatment is given in principle when an HIV infection is documented". They named a number of reasons that might restrict this indication, amongst them: "With high CD4 values (>500/mm$^3$) and low viral load (<5'000 RNA copies/ml), therapy can be delayed for the moment and further progression is monitored" (SKK/EKAF 1997: 20). The version of the guidelines that was updated December 21 1999 set the boundaries for treatment, which they also define as the boundaries indicating immune deficiency, at "CD4 >350/µl or viral load <5'000-30'000 copies/ml plasma"[112]. The very same guidelines, before being updated, used the same text with different boundaries, i.e. "CD4 >350-500/µl or viral load <5'000-10'000 copies/ml plasma". These changes in numbers, which are neither explicitly referred to nor explained in the guidelines[113], expand the range of laboratory values that justify deciding against treatment. Such changes are not trivial since the boundaries indicating treatment given in the guidelines have both a practical and a symbolic value. As the general practitioner Gregor Pfister noted, "this boundary becomes almost magical, and it is very much emotionally charged".

The changes in the Swiss guidelines over the short period of less than three years show that our study took place during a time of intense re-interpretations of the definition of HIV, AIDS, and its medical management. Two main developments characterize the changes in laboratory values. Firstly, the range of laboratory values justifying delaying treatment were gradually expanded, with CD4 cells dropping from 500 to 350-500 to 350/µl, and the viremia rising from <5'000 over <5'000-

---

[112] http://www.hivnet.ch/e/index-frame.html.

[113] In fact, I only became aware of the changes because I happened to print a version of the guidelines before the changes were made and consulted them again on the Internet after December 21, 1999.

10'000 to <5'000-30'000 copies/ml plasma. This development reflects the increasing skepticism about treating asymptomatic patients with favorable laboratory values. Secondly, in the case of the viremia, the guidelines also developed from indicating a clear-cut boundary, i.e. 5'000 copies/ml plasma, toward a widening range of values, covering first 5'000-10'000 and later 5'000-30'000 copies/ml plasma. The scope for autonomous decision-making of patients and physicians was thus gradually enlarged.

The clear-cut threshold values set mainly in the early versions of the guidelines reflect the desire to indicate measurable, comparable, objective boundaries, even if they are inevitably provisional and continuously shifting. Kaufert (1988) interpreted this widespread desire in medicine as an attempt to define boundaries to categorize patients and to cumulate research findings. Following DelVecchio Good (1995a), the certainty suggested by such recommendations may also be an attempt to compensate for the uncertainty about the long-term outcome of treatment, an outcome that remains, in the case of HIV, still unclear.

General practitioners and HIV specialists interpreted the changing recommendations given in the Swiss guidelines differently. The lower usage of antiretroviral treatment amongst HIV/AIDS patients in the general practice as compared to HIV centers indicate that general practitioners were already during our study in 1997 and early 1998 more inclined to what the United States guidelines soon after called "the therapeutically more cautious approach" (Feinberg 1998: 49). In the light of more cautious attitudes toward treatment receiving official status and the boundaries of the treatment-free area gradually being expanded, some of general practitioners' reluctance and skepticism against the wide implementation of antiretroviral treatment takes on a new meaning. What once was stubborn resistance against scientific evidence and progress foreshadowed a new trend and was to become mainstream.

When looking back with some retrospective distance, patients' decisions not to start treatment against the recommendations of physicians and guidelines are in some instances reinterpreted as wise decisions. As Luca Granges, an HIV specialist, said about his patient who had delayed treatment for a long time:

> "As a long-term survivor he remained skeptical for a long time. And he was probably right about it, as I must say retrospectively. I think he really judged it right when he did not start treatment, he probably would not have had any profit from it."

The skepticism concerning the use of antiretroviral therapies early in the infection that replaced the initial euphoria over having a possibility for action and the shifting emphasis on potential risks and adverse effects of treatment might follow a characteristic cycle of therapeutic innovations which was named by Fox (1980) as the "clinical moratorium". The clinical moratorium is, according to Fox, a marked slowdown in the use of a still-experimental form of a therapy, which can last for weeks, months, or years. Based upon empirical research in various medical fields, Fox described the "clinical moratorium" as a "recurrent, quasi-institutionalized event, most likely to take place during the early, 'black years' of the use of a new drug, device, or procedure with patient-subjects, when problems with uncertainty are especially salient and acute" (ibid.: 12). The skepticism can come from physician-researchers themselves, from their institutions or colleagues, from patients and their families. Placing the growing skepticism toward the broad use of HIV combination therapies into the context of medical history, the movement from "euphoria" towards "new realism" thus seems in the light of the clinical moratorium neither a new nor a surprising phenomenon. It might have been anticipated by patients and general practitioners who practiced realism while scientists and specialists were still overwhelmed by euphoria.

# CHAPTER 5

# FIGHTING OVER PATIENTS AND POWER

## MARKUS MADER: FROM MY WORM'S-EYE VIEW

I have gone through special stories with her. She came to me with this diagnosis, inflammation of the middle ear, and she said that she tried to cure it with a homeopathic treatment. And yet she came to an orthodox physician, she was very reserved, but in a border zone: Shall I go on as I did, or shall I treat it according to orthodox medicine? It was quite difficult. When I have patients like her, I try not to take their decision off their shoulders, but to give them the bases in order to allow them to decide by themselves. That's my attitude. I rarely decide for the patients, but I tell them that quite directly.

Orthodox medicine is a second and easily accessible option to her, an option that she would use, that she actually has been using since she has that disease. But on the other hand I realized that I strongly support the side in her that says: I am healthy, I can look after myself, and I move independently of this huge apparatus and system. I think this is not such a bad idea, also considering the history of medicine. I might have to say that I also did research. In the beginning of my career I did a lot of work on infectious diseases, a thesis on it, for a year I looked at post-antibiotic effects, and for a while I even wanted to become a specialist in infectious diseases. I have a long story there, quite special. But after my further education in the practice I moved very far away from orthodox medicine. I can look at it from a distance. Over the years I became quite critical and I got to see a lot of damage, iatrogenic damage through medicine. And partly it wasn't even caused by pharmacological aspects, but also through physician's behavior and communication. There were for example people who became suicidal through statements given by physicians from a clinic. I must say that's absolutely catastrophic.

The most important thing to me is the meaning that sickness has for the individual person in his environment. After all, what the patient is looking for in consultation is some kind of a perspective for health and for life. Of course there are also people who would like to receive a rather patriarchal type of guidance. They say: you are the doctor. When I give them the choice for one or the other thing and I say it would make sense to treat it in this way, then they say: well, you are the doctor, you have to decide. I answer: yes, of course, I am the doctor, but I am not going to swallow these tablets, you will have to swallow them, and that's why you have to know if you can do it.

Whenever I had HIV patients that took treatment, they all came to you[114], to the clinic. I know X, the senior physician, very well. Health care was shared. The general practitioner's access to knowledge is...– I think you need a specialist when treatment is required. If a patient really decides for it, then he must be in the care of someone who really has the routine down. On the whole, it actually works well. What I think is a pity is that on your side there are certain inconsistencies. In medicine, coherence in care is currently so miserable that I think we first have to check our own structures before we talk about patients. There would be quite some work to do. That's why I am active in the field of Quality Management in Family Practice. Total Quality Management means that everybody who participates in a process is involved in the improvement of this process. Of course the patient is the most important person in this process, and that's often forgotten in our care net.

Actually the basic structure of care, with specialized clinics where we can send people, is all right. To me they are like assistants for special tasks. But what I often find difficult is that it becomes unclear who finally is responsible for patient care; often the patient himself doesn't know who looks after what anymore. My experience is that orthodox medicine is often so much case-oriented and lacks continuity that over the years the scientific approach may be given, but the rest that our clinical medicine offers to the patient and that might be important for him is catastrophic. That's why we have patients who say: I am never going there again, no matter what you say. We clearly need a better flow of information, also from our side, and the acknowledgement that continuity must be the general practitioner's responsibility who can ensure it for a longer time.

I have seen strange stories. People come into my practice and something is prescribed, and then they come to the clinic and they simply prescribe a new package, without asking if we already started, just really confusing things. From my perspective as a general practitioner concerning collaboration, I would suggest to the insurance companies not to pay things like that anymore. If a hospital is not capable of consulting the general practitioner and starting a treatment concept by first looking at what has been done before, then it should not be financed anymore. Simply boycott them. And on the general practitioners' side exactly the same: if they don't learn to collaborate in a clearly defined way, then simply stop collaborating with them. This is exactly what the patients are currently doing instead of the physicians, and that's a pity, because it may be to the disadvantage of the patient.

When I work with the center, part of my role is to translate to the patient what I receive as a report. You at the clinic tend to be quite well behaved in doing that, with a list of problems and so on. It is my task to bring all that somehow together and to see what the whole care means to the patient and how he experiences it. And maybe there my impressions might be right that the patient's experience is, at least from my worm's-eye view, and from my outside perspective, not so positive. Even when everything looks like a lot and very comprehensive, somehow it is meager, patients lack the perspective that they feel understood and helped. And then with my information I more or less have to build up the whole thing and make it meaningful again. I think the patient often needs someone who checks with him if he really understood things. Somehow like an outside perspective, and sometimes also, so to speak, after he went through the whole apparatus.

---

[114] Through our institutional affiliation with the HIV clinic, my colleague and I were, as mentioned in chapter 1, to some degree associated with it. In the case of Markus Mader, this association may have been strengthened since for the interview he chose to come to our office at the clinic.

Continuity is essential if long-term care is to remain helpful. If the general practitioner drops out, then it is... – well, I must say, I mainly experience the negative effects. There are for example patients who suddenly come back into consultation, crying, and they have gone through a patient career without ever having had the opportunity to reflect with someone what would actually be important. They get into such an apparatus, and what they lack is a critical overview. It is absolutely invaluable if you built up trustworthiness in the doctor-patient interaction over time. This is so important for everything to come that I think it is the greatest potential to heal someone. But currently orthodox medicine does not acknowledge this importance. Medicine rather seems to work reparative, so to speak. When I now, after some ten years, look at the reports of such a clinic, they are sometimes ridiculous to look at retrospectively after four, five years. What does it mean in the life of a patient what a clinician or a team found? It is so relative. And that's why the long-term perspective is much more profound.

*\*\*\**

Combination therapies redefine the roles, work, authority, and competence of general practitioners and HIV specialists as well as the interaction between them. While in Switzerland medical specialists generally gain importance in health care, this process is much more accentuated in the case of HIV/AIDS where general practitioners are becoming increasingly excluded from the knowledge on treatment and the claim to integrate their HIV patients into specialized clinics and to "share" (Orton 1994) their care with specialists becomes stronger. The interaction at the generalist-specialist interface in HIV/AIDS therefore receives new importance as well as new potential for conflict. This process partly reflects developments taking place also in other areas of health care, and partly it might foreshadow them. In the present chapter, I present three patterns of allocating orthodox health care as emerging in our study: health care shared between general practitioners and HIV specialists, health care provided exclusively by the general practitioner and health care provided exclusively by the HIV specialist. I focus on the allocation of roles and, where applicable, the interaction between general practitioners and specialists as they were intensely debated, negotiated, and in the process of (re-)definition during our empirical research.

## 5.1. STRUGGLES AT THE INTERFACE

The discussion around the roles and collaboration of generalists and specialists has been most vividly led in Great Britain where schemes for "shared care" between general practitioners and specialists have been developed for a number of mainly chronic diseases (Grun and Murray 1995). The arguments that have been given in favor of primary care include accessibility, flexibility, comprehensiveness, cost-effectiveness, and a higher potential for an on-going doctor-patient relationship (Lewis 1997; Mansfield and Singh 1993; Orton 1994; Wigersma et al. 1998). Unlike other diseases where the general practitioner in Great Britain generally acts as a portal of entry ("gatekeeper") to specialized care (Orton 1994) and thus has a stronger position than in Switzerland, people with HIV have been encouraged to use Genito-Urinary Medicine clinics for both their primary and specialist care, resulting in little involvement of general practitioners in HIV care (Clarke 1993; Huby et al. 1998; Sheldon et al. 1993). Shared care schemes to increase the involvement of general practitioners into the care of HIV-positive patients have been implemented with limited success (Grun and Murray 1995; Madge et al. 1998).

With the advent of antiretroviral combination therapies, shared care schemes and efforts to enhance the involvement of the general practitioner in HIV care in order to increase accessibility and comprehensiveness became more controversially discussed and to some extent replaced by a new concern over treatment competence. A whole body of articles and editorials that discussed the allocation of care after the spread of combination therapies indicated that medical care provision for HIV patients became "an issue under intense debate" (Lewis 1997: 1133). Given the increasingly complex therapies (Feinberg 1998), it was argued that specialized physicians best manage HIV, although acknowledging that specialists may also include experienced and well-trained general practitioners. Zuger and Sharp explicitly challenged earlier efforts toward involving general practitioners in HIV care: "The 'primary care' algorithms of the early 1990s, in which asymptomatic persons were largely candidates for health monitoring rather than medical intervention, now seem quite outdated" (1997: 1131).

The discussion around the allocation of HIV care in the era of combination therapies was and still is redefining HIV care as the domain of specialists and experts. The arguments brought forward center around a discourse of competence expressed through experience with HIV. Practically all authors entering the debate refer to a study linking survival of male patients with AIDS to the experience of their primary care physicians (Kitahata et al. 1996)[115]. A second study often cited to support the claim for specialized HIV care stated that primary care physicians frequently miss important physical findings related to HIV infection during patient examination (Paauw et al. 1995). All of these studies were conducted before the introduction of antiretroviral treatment and exclusively involved symptomatic patients. Nevertheless, they serve as evidence to claim the care of asymptomatic patients as the specialist's domain, since these patients become candidates for complicated interventions, i.e. combination therapies. The argument is supported by the redefinition of HIV as a chronic treatable disease (see chapter 2.2.) which de-emphasizes the boundary between asymptomatic HIV infection (formerly seen as the legitimate domain of the generalist with a passive role of "monitoring") and symptomatic AIDS disease (as the domain of the expert with an active role of treat-

---

[115] A more recent study looking retrospectively at survival of female patients with AIDS between 1989-1992 found the same association for the latest study period from 1991 to 1992 (Laine et al. 1998).

ment and intervention): "Bisecting HIV disease into the simple, asymptomatic stage managed by the primary care clinician and the complex symptomatic stage requiring specialty consultation has become virtually obsolete" (Zuger and Sharp 1997: 1131)[116].

With antiretroviral treatment, the definition of expertise through "technical" skills including treatment administration and physical examinations thus tends to gain the upper hand over the "caring" aspects of comprehensiveness and a lasting doctor-patient interaction brought forward in favor of the general practitioner. Zuger and Sharp though did not only emphasize technical skills, but also used this very demand for comprehensive care to call for exclusive care through specialists. They described managed care models relying on shared care schemes as problematic since the specialist's consultative role remains "episodic and discontinuous" (ibid.: 1132), a problem that should be solved through exclusive care through specialists[117]. Specialization though, as they acknowledge, is not necessarily defined by the formation of the physician: "Scientifically and practically, HIV infection simply does not fit well into the neatly dichotomized boxes of 'general care' and 'specialty care'. (...) The truth is that many generalists have become, over the years, expert practitioners of HIV care. At the same time, many infectious disease specialists have remained both disinterested and inexpert. (...). AIDS should be the first disease for which the caricatures of 'consultant' and 'generalist' are finally retired and, instead, suitably qualified physicians are allowed and encouraged to provide all necessary facets of medical care" (ibid.: 1132). Soloway also questioned the boundaries between generalists and specialists: "The very concept of 'specialist' is a slippery one in the context of HIV. (...) no studies have demonstrated that the field in which a practitioner received formal training has an impact on the quality of care or outcome" (1997: 40). Though departing from a similar perspective as Zuger and Sharp, Soloway contrasts them by advocating a strong position of family physicians: "Do these concerns place treatment of HIV infection beyond the ability of family physicians and other primary care physicians? Hundreds of primary care practitioners, including many family physicians, have already demonstrated the contrary by successfully incorporating state-of-the-art antiviral therapies into their practices" (ibid.: 41).

---

[116] Abandoning this bisection between HIV and AIDS follows what Whittaker (1992) in the early 1990s already described as a counter-discourse of people with HIV constructing the infection as a continuum with the possibility of reversal through action.

[117] In blaming managed care systems for discontinuous specialist care, Zuger and Sharp name structures beyond the physician's sphere of competence as causing the problematic situation. Their argument thus is paralleled by an implicit argument against a current tendency to shift power beyond the medical domain toward health managers who establish care models that put physicians into a position where they are "forced by terms of their employment into a choice between a strictly consultative or primary care practice" (1997: 1132). See also chapters 5.2. and 6.7. on the economic structures of health care.

As the above arguments illustrate, creating HIV as a disease continuum and expanding the boundary of treatment toward the early phases of the infection is directly linked to the question of who is allowed or defined as competent to care for and treat HIV patients. The evocative style ("A New Era in HIV Care"[118]) and polemic claims ("'HIV Specialists': The Time Has Come"[119]) do not only reproduce the big phrases used by basic scientists promoting these therapies ("Time to Hit HIV, Early and Hard"[120]), but also indicate how much is at stake for physicians fighting over patients and power. Lewis (1997: 1134) reasoned with the very "hit early and hard" approach of basic science when discussing the United States guide-lines on antiretroviral treatment issued in 1997: "What is now being proposed by some is to limit the role of most primary care physicians to that of screening and diagnosis, and then either referring to or establishing a contact with an 'AIDS expert' to plan a program of therapy. This is especially true as the 'hit early and hard' approach to antiretroviral treatment is now widely accepted by many leaders in the field". The 1998 United States guidelines claimed that "treatment of HIV-infected patients should be directed by a physician with extensive experience in the care of these patients. When this is not possible, the physician treating the patient should have access to such expertise through consultations" (Feinberg 1998). While exper-tise and experience thus stand at the core of the physician's qualification for treat-ment, also the guidelines carefully seem to omit an allocation of expertise to HIV specialists, thus trying to stay off the turf battles between generalists and specialists over HIV care. The Swiss guidelines (SKK/EKAF 1997; 1998) which largely tend to follow the United States guidelines are more explicit in allocating expertise by sug-gesting that general practitioners should collaborate with a specialized HIV center.

It is generally acknowledged that expertise includes also experienced and trained general practitioners, i.e. it does not necessarily run along institutional boundaries like HIV clinics or along the formal qualifications of the physician: The inclusion of "suitably qualified" (Zuger and Sharp 1997: 1132) general practitioners into the definition of HIV/AIDS experts though does not threaten the domain of HIV spe-cialists since it is commonly argued that most general practitioners have too few patients to become experts (Lewis 1997). As our data indicate for the example of Switzerland, it is indeed only a small minority of general practitioners which is experienced in HIV in terms of caring for a larger number of HIV patients (Figure 13).

---

[118] As Soloway (1997) titled his claim for a strong position of family practitioners in HIV care.

[119] As Zuger and Sharp (1997) titled their claim for HIV as an infection requiring specialized care.

[120] As Ho (1995) titled his claim for early treatment of HIV with combination therapy. See also chapter 2.3..

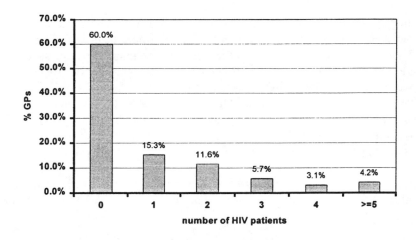

*Figure 13. Number of HIV patients per general practitioner*

As shown earlier in table 12 and figure 6, many people with HIV were under care at a general practitioner's, and general practitioners were chosen more frequently with a prolonged duration of the infection. Nevertheless, only 40.0% of the general practitioners in our sample cared for HIV patients. This percentage is comparable to the one found in a study among general practitioners in the Swiss canton Berne conducted in 1989 where 32% of the general practitioners had HIV patients (Malinverni et al. 1992). Many general practitioners in our sample had only one (15.3%) or two (11.6%) HIV patients, and only 4.2% of all general practitioners had five or more HIV patients, with the upper limit at 65 patients per practitioner. Only a minority of general practitioners is therefore experienced in HIV in terms of more frequent patient care. The 4.2% (n=23) of general practitioners with five or more HIV patients united 46.6% (n=321) of the total of 691 HIV patients under care at the general practitioners in our sample. This concentration of HIV patients around a relatively small segment of general practitioners was even more pronounced than in the study from 1989 by Malinverni et al. (1992) where 8% of the general practitioners from the city and suburbs of Berne cared for one third of all HIV patients. A similar clustering of a high number of HIV patients around a small number of general practitioners was also found in a Dutch study where the 16 general practitioners from Amsterdam participating in the study cared for more than one third of all people with HIV/AIDS in Amsterdam (Redijk et al. 1999).

The concentration of a high number of HIV/AIDS patients around a relatively small number of general practitioners indicates that while most general practitioners are inexperienced with HIV, many HIV patients are under care at more experienced general practitioners (if experience is defined in terms of numbers of HIV/AIDS patients). The majority of HIV patients were under care at their general practitioner without additional care provided by an HIV clinic: More than half (53.1%) of the 691 HIV/AIDS patients under care at the general practitioners in our sample were not additionally under care at an HIV center (see also chapter 4.1.). Also in the era of combination therapies, it thus remained more common for general practitioners in Switzerland to care for HIV patients without collaborating with the specialized HIV clinics. From our data, the reasons against collaboration can only be hypothesized. Firstly, some of the general practitioners not sharing care with a center may indeed have the expertise experienced general practitioners are granted in the controversy over allocating HIV care and they thus may not require specialist consultation. Secondly, some of the general practitioners (or their patients) may "resolve problems that occur at the primary-secondary interface" (King et al. 1998: 1236) simply by omitting that interface.

Amongst the general practitioners who had patients which were additionally under care at an HIV center, a majority of 74.9% rated the collaboration with the center as good (table 18). This high percentage indicates that, if care was indeed shared between general practitioners and HIV clinics, general practitioners commonly viewed it as positive. Shared care therefore has a good potential to combine in the care of the individual patient the different aspects of health care as provided by physicians of different institutional and educational background. On the other hand, 25.1% of general practitioners found the collaboration with the HIV center to be difficult.

*Table 18. Collaboration with the HIV center*

|           | n   | %     |
|-----------|-----|-------|
| Good      | 131 | 74.9  |
| Difficult | 44  | 25.1  |
| Total     | 175 | 100.0 |

When asked about the types of difficulties in collaboration with the HIV center, 31 of the general practitioners named lack of information from the center, 25 found that the center took over the work of the general practitioner, and 18 criticized that the center didn't discuss its interventions with the general practitioner (table 19).

*Table 19. Problems in collaborating with the HIV center*

|                                          | n  | %     |
|------------------------------------------|----|-------|
| Information flow                         | 31 | 70.5  |
| HIV center replaces GP                   | 25 | 56.8  |
| HIV center doesn't discuss               | 18 | 40.9  |
| interventions with GP                    |    |       |
| Other                                    | 6  | 13.6  |
|                                          | 44 | 100.0 |

The literature on the subject generally describes and constructs the interface between generalists and specialists as an area of tension. Clarke (1993) found a less than optimal level of communication between hospital services, patients, and general practitioners, and Mansfield and Singh (1993) stated that poor communication between specialists and general practitioners has become institutionalized. There are different approaches suggested to resolve these tensions. As outlined above, some researchers favor approaches that omit the interaction between generalists and specialists by entirely relocating HIV care to the specialist. In contrast, Huby et al. (1998) discussed the general practitioners' relative lack of contact with other service providers found in their study ("general practitioners saw people, but in isolation", ibid.: S86) as corresponding to some of their patients' expectations: "the general practitioner-patient relationship was valued for being familiar and on-going. It appeared that people valued their relationship with their general practitioner precisely because it was peripheral to the hospital-based system of information exchange, evaluation and control" (ibid.: S86). Researchers in favor of shared care unanimously call for improved communication and collaboration between generalists and specialists. King et al. (1998) demanded improved information between caregivers, Wigersma et al. (1998), Madge et al. (1998), and Orton (1994) rated the collaboration between primary care, secondary care, and the affected community as a major prerequisite for accessible and comprehensive care.

## 5.2. KNOWLEDGE IS POWER IS MONEY

The collaboration between general practitioners and specialists at the HIV centers cannot be reduced to practical problems, such as organizing a smooth flow of information or allocating responsibilities when planning interventions, for it involves an asymmetrical relationship. Although general practitioners with a private practice are institutionally independent, they may depend on the knowledge of specialists, especially knowledge concerning treatment, in the care of their patients. The knowledge asymmetry between general practitioners and specialists in clinics has a potential to create tension and conflicts, as expressed most vividly by Gregor Pfister:

"We general practitioners are not all that stupid. But sometimes that's what the HIV clinics make us feel like. Sure, they have specialized knowledge, but we all used to work in clinics."

In his statement, Gregor Pfister refers to hierarchy of knowledge[121] in medicine, with specialized knowledge claiming a higher position than the knowledge of the general practitioner who may in the interaction with the specialist feel "stupid". Gregor Pfister located the source of specialized knowledge in the clinic, thus lying partly beyond his reach as general practitioner and therefore providing an explanation for the disparaging behavior of the specialist. Yet the argument that "we all used to work in clinics" also de-emphasizes the boundary between generalists and specialists and thus questions the justification of the asymmetry by pointing out the personal link of general practitioners whose biography as physicians and whose personal competence is rooted in clinics. Similarly, in the narrative introducing the present chapter, Markus Mader underlined his competence by relating to his experience with clinical research in the field of infectious diseases.

Turner described a mutual relationship between medical knowledge, medical dominance, and the clinic: in modernity, expanding medical knowledge and domination developed hand in hand and are in turn accompanied by the growth and specialization of clinics as the principal settings of medical technology and practice. The clinic became the symbol and focal point of the growing dominance and professional power of medicine in society (Foucault 1996; Turner 1995).

Given that "{u}nprecedented advances in the biosciences and medical technologies characterize our contemporary world" (DelVecchio Good 1995a: 205), specialized medicine, and the clinic as a major source of it, currently gain further terrain at the expense of general medicine. DelVecchio Good pointed out that the "turf battles" between generalists and specialists could thus be interpreted as a barometer of the developments in medical knowledge and techniques. In the case of HIV/AIDS, these developments have been greatly accelerated prior to our study through the introduction of a new diagnostic technique (measurement of viral load) and novel and successful therapeutic options (combination therapies including the new protease inhibitors). HIV/AIDS therefore provides an example of how changing knowledge in one specific field profoundly changes the roles of generalists and specialists as well as their interaction. The developments in the field of HIV/AIDS reproduce and perpetuate a broad process in medicine. Turner's observation that the fragmentation of the medical profession into specialists who control the medical profession and general practitioners whose position is deteriorating seems to be reflected by the situation in Switzerland. Within the ten years prior to our study, the

---

[121] As Herzlich reminded us, "medical knowledge, as actually used by a given practitioner, always takes us back to the physician's place in the entire medical institution" (1995:157).

share of physicians specialized in general medicine amongst the physicians approved by the Swiss Medical Association FMH which are working in a practice dropped from 25.2% (n=2163) in 1988 to 19.0% (n=2505) in 1998 while the total number of physicians increased (Generalsekretariat der Verbindung der Schweizer Ärztinnen und Ärzte FMH 1999; Verbindung der Schweizer Ärzte 1988). Looking at the percentages of physicians newly approved by the Swiss Medical Association hints at the future of general medicine: in 1998, merely 8.3% (n=67) of all the new FMH titles were achieved in the field of general medicine. Percentages of physicians specialized in general medicine are also decreasing in other countries: In France for example, the share of general practitioners dropped from two thirds in 1980 to half of all physicians in 1997 (Rondeau 1999).

The decreasing overall income of physicians diagnosed by the Swiss Medical Association (Brunner 1997b) is mainly characterized by the income gap between generalists and specialists. Narrowing that gap is one of the central goals of the general revision of the medical tariffs in Switzerland through a project initially named "Gesamtrevision Arzttarif"[122] GRAT and subsequently renamed to TarMed. Increasing the generalists' income should be achieved through better compensation for "basic services" as opposed to "operative services" and the use of technical equipment. In the early versions of the GRAT, basic services were referred to as "intellectual services" in opposition to "technical services". Specialists, providing a higher share of "technical services" and thus fearing for their income, perceived this terminology as degrading. As a surgeon asked on the homepage of the Swiss Medical Association: "Would it mean that a surgeon does not use his intelligence when operating?"[123].

Along with concerns over the loss of the profession's autonomy through external interference into the tariffs (see chapter 6.7.), the fight between generalists and specialists over income distribution has been and still is the focal point of the emotional debates around the project TarMed. "Hysteria increasingly seems to replace a rational discourse", as the president of the Swiss Medical Association was cited (Trutmann and Steiner 1999). Surgeons are on the forefront of the opposition against the new tariffs which they believe to decrease their income by an average of 43% (Ritschard 2000). In the eyes of a physician cited on the homepage of the Swiss Medical Association, economic factors received such an importance in drawing the boundary between specialists and generalists that he viewed the division between them as actually being *produced* by the revision of tariffs. The same physician also believed the loss of physicians' professional autonomy to be a consequence

---

[122] General revision of physicians' tariffs

[123] www.fmh.ch/d/tarmed, January 18, 2000

of this very division: "The division between generalists and specialists was produced by GRAT and surrendered the medical profession to bureaucracy"[124].

### 5.3. WHO CURES? WHO CARES?

Ultimately, the concrete object fought for in the struggles between generalists and specialists is the patient, being the content of work, the legitimization, and the source of income for the physician. Discussions around the respective roles of generalists and specialists in HIV care may culminate into the question of who "owns" the patient, a question that Clarke (1993) also found to be discussed amongst health care providers in England. Different actors may have contradictory notions of the respective roles of specialists and generalists in patient care. The statements of the HIV specialist Luca Granges and the general practitioner Gregor Pfister show how they may clash:

> "The patient was referred to us by the general practitioner and I took him over from my predecessor. (...). When I took him over, the decision concerning treatment was due, and we discussed the pros and cons for quite a long time. Then we started therapy, and it was clear that in the framework of the study protocol more blood tests were necessary, and therefore he simply came here. And when we became aware of any other problems because we had to fill them into the study protocol, it turned out that for smaller problems I more or less took over the role of a general practitioner." (Luca Granges)

> "We have to rely on the collaboration with the center. I also think it makes sense that the indication for medication, which is after all also expensive, comes from the center. But of course it is not possible that the patient then receives primary care through the outpatient department, since this is just exactly non-care. I do not get the information on what happens and the patient doesn't really know anymore, especially with minor things, if he should refer to the center or to me for them, and he is not quite integrated anymore. I have several of these patients. (...). A physician from a center[125] clearly stated to me that their maxim was: we take the patients to us and away from the general practitioner. The center in X denies that, they say, no, that is not their goal, but that is what it comes down to." (Gregor Pfister)

Mansfield and Singh (1993) found in England that specialists may indeed replace primary care physicians when they are expected to support them. In the struggle over patients, generalist and specialists use different strengths and strategies. As noted in chapter 3.4., specialists gained back the competence of curing through antiretroviral treatment; with the new emphasis on curing, the caring aspects of their work – which had inevitably been more central as long as there was no "cure" to offer – lost some of its importance and some of its problems. This new accent, generally welcomed with relief by specialists, may also have the consequence that the specialist's role becomes narrowed and reduced to the curing

---

[124] www.fmh.ch/d/tarmed, January 18, 2000

[125] Gregor Pfister does not refer to the center where the specialist Luca Granges, cited above, works.

aspects. Andreas Bauer described his new role as that of a "technician", implying that with antiretroviral treatment some of the skills he formerly used in his work became obsolete. He though emphasized that the role of the "technician" also demands new skills on the caring side of his work since treatment creates new problems:

> "Health care changed a lot. A few years ago, we treated complications when they appeared, or we tried to prevent them. Nowadays there are barely any complications left, and we became technicians of antiretroviral therapy. The problem is not necessarily less complicated, nor less interesting or complex, that's clear, since there is now the whole side of adherence to treatment, patient support, psychological support in accepting treatment, support in taking treatment regularly, explaining, re-explaining, etc.. Things really did change, but they are not less interesting, rather the contrary."
> (Andreas Bauer)

It seems that specialists may compensate the possibility of becoming excluded from the caring, the „human" side of medical work through emphasizing the caring aspects required to ensure continuous treatment adherence. The demand for and the problems of adherence thus allow relocating to some degree the caring aspects into treatment and thus into the domain of the specialists. While specialists become "therapy technicians", often taking over the role of merely initiating and changing treatment when sharing care with a general practitioner, generalists have to reflect on *their* role under the new condition. Sharing care between general practitioner and specialist (Orton 1994), as suggested also in the Swiss HIV treatment guidelines (SKK/EKAF 1998), means that the general practitioner becomes both integrated into the care and treatment schemes of HIV clinics yet excluded from the competence of curing. Both of these aspects may be problematic to some of the general practitioners. On the one hand, integration into clinical care may be, as noted above, not only difficult to organize and involve an asymmetrical relationship, but it may also stand in opposition to the very reason why some patients choose the general practitioner, i.e. for the continuous care relation with a single physician. On the other hand, exclusion from treatment might question the competence of the general practitioner to a point that s/he becomes ignored or obsolete in patient care.

The general practitioner has two possibilities to deal with these processes of both structural inclusion into clinical care and exclusion from treatment competence. Firstly, s/he can choose to remain outside the clinic-based system. The importance of this strategy might be reflected by the fact that more than half of all patients with antiretroviral treatment from our sample of general practitioners are not "shared" with the center. Secondly, s/he can accentuate and elaborate his/her competence in other aspects of patient care. As commonly argued in the literature on shared care, the role and competence of the general practitioner lies in organizing comprehensive and continuous care and assuring through an ongoing doctor-patient relationship that the patients' view is elicited and integrated into health care (Orton 1994). This role is indeed stressed by many general practitioners when defining their work.

Markus Mader for example distinguishes in the narrative introducing this chapter the role of the specialist and the generalist mainly through the temporal dimension of their work: The specialist is needed for selective short-term interventions while the general practitioner ensures long-term coherence of care. By stressing that the long-term perspective is more important in the biography of a patient, he emphasized the aspect of patient care that favors the general practitioner as more important. François Neher summarized the focus on caring in the work of the general practitioner as follows:

> "I believe that our purpose as physicians is to be guided by the patient's wishes."
> (François Neher)

As negotiated and articulated in the field of HIV/AIDS, the general practitioner's and the specialist's role in health care are gradually becoming more distinguished from each other. While the generalist ensures that the patient's wishes are integrated into health care, the specialist assumes responsibility and competence over treatment. Increasing efforts for collaboration between generalists and specialists do not stand in opposition to such a division of labor, but rather are the precondition for it. Only through such a division is either side allowed to concentrate primarily on their respective aspect of patient care. In an HIV clinic, Silverman and Bloor found a Cartesian division of labor between physicians and psychological counselors where "doctors take bodies and counselors take minds" (1990: 10). The collaboration between general practitioner and specialist and their division of labor in patient care might ultimately lead into a similar division of the patient, with the patient as "person" assigned to the general practitioner and the patient as "body" to the specialist. While specialized medicine perfects the clinical gaze on and into the body, extracts data from it through its technology and in return alters its functioning through the input of medication, general medicine guides the person through this process according to his/her preferences and attitudes. In that sense, the division of labor between physicians and psychological counselors described by Silvermann and Bloor might increasingly be reproduced *within* the medical profession between specialists and generalists.

# CHAPTER 6

# EVIDENCE VS. EXPERIENCE

"Distrust of science is still alarmingly prevalent, which conflicts with reasonable expectations. Is not the century now drawing to a close most of all remarkable for the technology that now fills our world and for the understanding of that world that has been won since, say, the discovery of the electron in 1897?" (Maddox 1995: 435)

## LUCA GRANGES: TWENTY YEARS FROM NOW WE MIGHT BE JUDGED

It started in fall when the results of this clinical trial became more and more clear. I counseled him, and since he decided to start treatment and became a participant in a study protocol, he has been exclusively in my care. If it was his wish to start treatment? Well, that's a bit difficult to say: his wish. There are guidelines. As far as anti-retroviral treatment is concerned, everything is changing incredibly fast. By the end of '95 we really had a breakthrough where you now see for the first time that this combination of two medicines has finally, after such a long time, shown a real improvement in survival. According to the guidelines at that time, he had no clear indication for treatment, where you had to say: okay, the viral load is so high and the helper cells are so low that you have to do something. But we have actually become more and more aggressive lately, over the last year.

There is this scientific evidence, there are studies showing this and that benefit, and then there is the question of how you can apply these findings to the individual patient. And there you always have discrepancies; you have to consider psychological and social moments, compliance and so on. But I have to say that back then we discussed this decision several times. It was a process lasting several weeks, maybe two or three months, if I remember correctly.

That he eventually stopped treatment was a very unhappy and strange story. He came into this protocol with a good combination therapy, although it did not contain protease inhibitors, and the first data of this study were promising. When the protocol was written, protease inhibitors were not yet on the market, they were in the process of approval. But I think it was a good therapy, and he responded well to it. Massive rise of helper cells, relevant virus suppression, everything worked perfectly, but then he

123

developed these side effects. That also worried me personally, it is exactly the most unpleasant situation, if you have people who feel well and start treatment with the idea of a long-term benefit, and then they develop side effects. It is the last thing you would want to happen.

We discussed the possibility of changing the medication combination, and now everything remains open. We thought it would be best to wait a bit. It was very important for him that he could go on vacation, which I understood very well. And he will go now. It was not an emergency case. He will come back after vacation and we will reassess the situation, and he has already expressed the wish to start another treatment. With these side effects I understood that he had had enough for the moment and wanted a certain distance. After all, it is not an easy decision, also whether to make a double or a triple combination. The idea that, since he has responded well to treatment so far, a double combination might be enough made him think quite a lot. But I must say now, also with these new guidelines, and with these results we have – I believe that he will start a triple combination.

There are so many things to consider... If you look for example at the whole story of tuberculosis; in the case of tuberculosis treatment, the "hit early and hard" approach makes sense. On the other hand, especially with this patient who responded so well to this first attempt, you might say we start just with a double combination, it is much easier to take and has fewer side effects. It is a difficult decision, especially since there is no clear evidence where you could say: "Look, this is what you have to do, this is the best thing". If someone has side effects from treatment but no symptoms from the HIV infection, it is a big burden to regularly take this medication. The decision is not so easy; it is a discretionary decision.

After all, it always depends on the patient if he really wants it. He is the one who decides, and not us – well, us too, because we are the specialists who can say how to set the course in a serious situation and when something has to be changed. But it always is the patient who plays the main part: his convictions, his motivation and his willingness. If someone says, although treatment is clearly indicated, he doesn't want it, then we don't do it, I don't do it. I clearly tell people that it is a far-reaching decision, and I also tell them: if you start something, you should see it through.

We still know far too little about combination therapies. But my impression is, also from what other people say, for example Margaret Fischl, whom I remember very well from the last AIDS meeting in Vancouver: with this medication we simply change the whole pool of virus. Sometime twenty years from now we might be judged and people might shake their heads about the nonsense we did. I certainly hope not.

***

With the rapid development of new antiretroviral therapies at the time of our empirical research, the transfer of knowledge and information from medical science to medical practice received new significance. New therapies were tested in clinical trials whose results were rapidly translated into new guidelines. The role of medical science and guidelines was discussed not only on a practical level, as physicians were struggling to acquire up to date information, but also on an ideological level. The questions of what types of knowledge are relevant to medical practice, who has the power and legitimacy to define this relevance, who produces relevant knowledge, how this knowledge is diffused and how it is applied in medical practice became controversially discussed.

In the present chapter, I explore the attempts to further integrate medical science into medical practice, the claims to standardize and control medical practice through these attempts, and the resistance against them. In the case of HIV, treatment guidelines as the most obvious symbol for the attempt to shape decision-making in medical practice, both in terms of how treatment is decided on as well as who should make these decisions, provide a focal point for these issues. On the broader level, a key term around which these issues are grouped and which I chose as a paradigm to discuss them is "Evidence-Based Medicine". In the definition of its founders, "{t}he practice of evidence-based medicine means integrating individual clinical experience with the best available external clinical evidence from systematic research" (Sackett et al. 1997: 2). Evidence-Based Medicine with its concern for basing clinical practice on scientific evidence in turn represents a new incarnation of a much older struggle over the meaning of "art" and "science" in medicine.

## 6.1. SCIENCE AND ART

"Science" and "art" are prominent and widely used metaphors to describe the tensions inherent to the work of the physician. They refer to two ideal and symbolically opposed types of medical knowledge to be combined in patient care: "science" produced by basic research and clinical trials on the one hand, medical expertise and experience[126] as the "art" of the individual physician on the other hand. The two models represent two different, idealized forms of knowledge: science being explicit, universal, and abstract, art being the personal knowledge of the physician acquired through and applied in the interaction with the individual patient. While it is acknowledged that science is subject to external review, art is seen as the implicit, tacit, "private magic" of a physician (Gordon 1988).

The description of the physician's work through science and art and the discussion of their conflicting relationship can be traced back to Greek philosophy. According to Wieland (1993), the concept of "art" did not have the modern aesthetic connotation. Instead, it represented in accordance with the Latin *ars* and the Greek

---

[126] Wieland defined medical experience as situated and personal, contrasting it to the abstract experience obtained in the experimental sciences: "The experimental sciences are concerned with supporting or rejecting general laws. The data of experience that contribute to this process are ideally simple, verifiable, and repeatable. In contrast, medical experience does not aim at general principles; it manifests itself in the physician's ability to evaluate correctly difficult and problematic individual facts and events. It is such experience that enables the physician to frame appropriate basic statements. It correlates with a disposition that is closely bound to the person of the physician. It cannot be separated from the person and transmitted directly" (1993: 175-176).

*techne* the human capacity for production by planned action, thus primarily representing an antithesis to nature. Aristotle further narrowed the concept of art by delimiting it from science (*episteme*). While science looks for universal laws, art as concrete action is directed toward the individual. Aristotle concluded that there is a fundamental tension between the two concepts, since art in its individual variety can never fully be grasped and formalized through science. This tension was exemplified by Aristotle through the very example of the physician whose work cannot entirely be guided by science since it is directed toward the individual patient.

Until the eighteenth century, the distinction between art and science did, according to Wieland, not have any polemical power, since medicine was a discipline based on a closed, dogmatic science which did not conflict with or question medical practice. Only with the development of an open, progressing science, the mediation between scientific findings and medical practice and thus the Aristotelian distinction between science and art became problematic and controversially discussed. While some hoped that the art of medicine would eventually be formalized as a science, others claimed that medicine should reserve areas in which science could not intrude.

The discussions held in the eighteenth and nineteenth century remarkably resemble the contemporary discussions of the conflicts the physician is confronted with in his/her practice. For many years, basic science moved into the laboratory to develop its theory, leaving care decisions to the individual physician whose work remained relatively unchallenged and without the reach of external evaluation (Gordon 1988). Over the last decades, clinical science as a link between basic science and medical practice was intensified. With the increasing importance of clinical science, paradigmatically represented through the double-blind controlled clinical trial, attempts are intensified to communicate research findings to the practicing physician and to base physicians' decision-making and practice on scientific evidence.

## 6.2. EVIDENCE-BASED MEDICINE

"Evidence-Based Medicine" is the master symbol for the further integration of medical science into the art of medicine. It tries to narrow the gap between research results and medical practice by supporting the physician in accessing and evaluating research results and applying them in practice. As Le Pen put it, Evidence-Based Medicine is "a philosophy, but it is also and above all a structured movement, a school, a journal, conferences, etc." (1999: 99). The term was coined in the 1980s at McMaster Medical School in Ontario, Canada, where Evidence-Based Medicine had been developed for over a decade as a clinical learning and problem-solving strategy. It is closely linked to the development and introduction of a new medical curriculum which involves abandoning traditional exams, introducing small studying groups supervised by a tutor, and problem-based learning strategies using Evidence-Based Medicine approaches (Chabot 1999; Rosenberg and Donald 1995). Evidence-Based Medicine tries to encourage and enable physicians to use three main strategies: "learning how to practice evidence-based medicine ourselves, seeking and applying evidence-based medical summaries produced by others and accepting evidence-based practice protocols developed by our colleagues and augmented by strategies that help us improve our clinical competence" (Sackett et al. 1997: 12). While the first of these strategies thus aims at training the physician in the new methods and approaches developed by Evidence-Based Medicine (such as performing systematic reviews and meta-analyses of clinical studies[127]), the second and third strategy aim at encouraging him/her to use the tools of Evidence-Based Medicine as developed by others. These tools include journals and databases publishing the results of systematic reviews and meta-analyses, evidence-based guidelines summarizing these findings, and individual feedback and advice by people trained in Evidence-Based Medicine. Practicing Evidence-Based Medicine means forming the relevant clinical questions, knowing how to search for the best external evidence and how to appraise that evidence for its validity and importance, how to apply it in practice and to evaluate one's own practical performance. This procedure may be applied to any sequence of medical work, starting from achieving a diagnosis and estimating a prognosis over deciding on therapy and determining its potential harm to providing care (Sackett et al. 1997).

Sackett and colleagues described the "progressive decline in our clinical competency after we complete our formal training"[128] (Sackett et al. 1997: 9) as a major reason for developing Evidence-Based Medicine. They – of course – support their statement by evidence which showed "repeatedly that there is a statistically and clinically significant negative correlation between our knowledge of up-to-date care and the years that have elapsed since our graduation from medical school"[129] (ibid.). In other words, the longer a physician has been practicing, the more s/he bases his/her work on obsolete knowledge. In order to challenge this dissatisfying situation, Evidence-Based Medicine outlines and teaches the skills and methods to formulate the relevant questions for a given problem, to search the literature for relevant articles, to evaluate the evidence provided in these articles for its validity and usefulness, and to implement valid and useful findings in practice (Ellrodt et al.

[127] See chapter 6.5. describing systematic reviews and meta-analyses as well as the media developed to publish them.
[128] Note the insistence on the inclusive "we" and "our", pronouns intended to bridge the gap between the proponents of Evidence-Based Medicine and medical practitioners by stressing their common identity as physicians.
[129] Note again the repeated "our".

1997; Rosenberg and Donald 1995). Such an approach is based on a model of competence that largely contracts common assumptions in medicine: the senior physician is usually seen as more competent than his/her junior colleagues precisely through the years elapsed since graduation, since s/he passed these years in medical practice and thus acquired vast experience. Sackett and colleagues instead emphasize the discrepancy between decisions based upon such experience and the latest findings of clinical science, and they interpret this discrepancy to the disadvantage of the senior physician.

Evidence-Based Medicine, co-developed and primarily represented by David Sackett from McMaster Medical School, is based upon clinical epidemiology. The subtitle of a book by Sackett and colleagues (1991) on clinical epidemiology, "A Basic Science for Clinical Medicine", is programmatic for the discipline. By its rigid, objective, and universally applicable methodology, clinical epidemiology is defined as a basic science (thus also claiming its prestige), yet its purpose and use lie in applied clinical medicine. The authors thus present their approach as a mediator between the distant, inaccessible sites of the production of medical knowledge and the everyday work of the notorious "busy clinicians" (Sackett and Cook 1994) sympathetically conjured up by Sackett and reproduced by his adherents (Rosenberg and Donald 1995). Correspondingly, the authors explicitly present "Clinical Epidemiology" "as a book for the 'users' of research done by others" (Sackett et al. 1991: x). In the book's preface, they describe their aim to explore the "science of the art of medicine" and thus to improve medical diagnosis, prognosis, management, learning and teaching. I quote the beginning of the book's preface at length, including also the paragraph in which David Sackett's (referred to as D.L.S.) biographical pathway towards clinical epidemiology is recounted:

> "*Clinical Epidemiology* has its origins in clinical practice, as we struggled with the diagnosis and management of our patients and fell slowly behind in our clinical reading. All of us had been trained in internal medicine, and all of us believed that we were practicing the Art (derived from the beliefs, judgments, and intuitions we could not explain), as well as the Science (derived from the knowledge, logic, and prior experience we could explain), of clinical medicine.
>
> At different times, and in different situations, it dawned on each of us that there was, in fact, a science to the art of medicine. For D.L.S., this realization came when the Cuban missile crisis transformed him, a tenderfoot nephrologist and renal tubular physiologist, into a reluctant field epidemiologist in the U.S. Public Health Service. Although obligated to learn epidemiology (most of it for the first time), he remained a clinician at heart and was repeatedly surprised by the extent to which his growing knowledge of epidemiologic principles could shed light both on the illnesses of patients and the diagnostic and management behavior of their clinicians. Moreover, it dawned on him that applying these epidemiologic principles (plus a few more from biostatistics) to the beliefs, judgments, and intuitions that comprise the art of medicine might substantially improve the accuracy and efficiency of diagnosis and prognosis, the effectiveness of management, the efficiency of trying to keep up to date, and, of special importance, the ability to teach others how to do these things. The opportunity to explore this sci-

ence of the art of medicine burgeoned with the creation of a new medical school at McMaster University, which D.L.S. joined in 1967 and where he later teamed up with the other authors to write up the first edition of this book." (Sackett et al. 1991: ix)[130]

The preface is noteworthy not only for its reference to art and science in medicine, but also for its introduction of the authors. Titled with "Origins", the authors create Evidence-Based Medicine's myth of foundation by speaking in the first person of their personal experience as medical practitioners in different "fields". By introducing their work with a personal narrative, they follow a common pattern to introduce ethnographic writing, as I mentioned in the introduction of this book[131] in referring to Pratt (1986). Although in a self-portrait considerably shorter[132] than commonly given by anthropologists, the parallels to ethnographic introductions go as far as including for example the customary use of irony. In fact, the personal and often humorous style that characterizes the writing by Sackett and colleagues (and pleasantly distinguishes it from most medical texts) might account for part of their success in medicine. Pratt holds that these "opening narratives" are not trivial, for they play the crucial role of anchoring the following formal, scientific part of the book in the intense and authority-giving personal experience. In the case of the introduction by Sackett, the narrative establishes the author both as an expert in the subject of his book as well as a physician facing the very problems his colleagues are struggling with.

Pratt found it noteworthy that the personal narrative persisted in scientific writing against academic pressure, which tended to devaluate it as mere anecdote. I find it all the more noteworthy when it is used by scientists who aim at preventing physicians from relying merely on personal experience and "beliefs" (which, according to Sackett and colleagues in the introduction cited above, belong to the art of medicine[133]), and who intend to limit the personal authority of experts[134]. The self-

---

[130] Copyright © 1991; *Little, Brown and Company*; reproduced here by kind permission of *Little, Brown and Company*.

[131] Where I, of course, try to accomplish through my own narrative similar effects as the ones outlined by Pratt.

[132] Shortness might typically distinguish medical from anthropological writing. DiGiacomo for example recounted how the anthropologist William Dressler, working with epidemiologists, described the epidemiologists' reaction to ethnography: "very nice, but so many words!" (1999: 449).

[133] The "belief" of physicians, as used in the cited preface, takes us back to the opposition on the "belief" and "knowledge" in medicine, as outlined in chapter 3.2. The attribution of "belief", commonly associated with the patient, to the physician highlights that approaches to control medical practice also involve a judgment of the physicians' knowledge as subjective. The subjectivity in medical practice though remains partial in the description of Sackett and colleagues for it is limited to the "art" of medical practice which ideally is complemented by the objectivity of medical science.

[134] To quote Sackett et al. on the quality of expert knowledge: "For example, the traditional review article, in which an 'expert' states opinions about the proper evaluation and management of a condition,

positioning both as experienced experts and "clinician at heart" might be, similarly as the repeated use of the pronouns "we" and "our", a strategy to deal with the delicacy of trying to interfere with the decision-making of the individual physician. In the face of physicians' resistance, trustworthiness and credibility have to be established, a task accomplished firstly by professional fraternization and secondly by claiming competence through experience, thus through the very factor otherwise described as an insufficient base for professional competence. The professional fraternization and creation of a common identity might be a strategy to compensate for Evidence-Based Medicine's criticism on medical work. On the one hand, it declares the criticism as coming from within medicine, thus neutralizing the notorious resistance of physicians against external critics. On the other hand, it implies that the proponents of Evidence-Based Medicine are confronted with the same problems as their colleagues whom they are criticizing.

## 6.3. THE VIEW FROM BELOW

Evidence-Based Medicine and its new emphasis on the problematic interaction of art and science in medicine turned into a prominent topic amongst physicians in the 1990s. The annual assembly of the Swiss Societies of General and of Internal Medicine in 1997 for instance was titled with "Primary Health Care: Science or Art?". In a speech held at the assembly, Fugelli feared an overdose of Evidence-Based Medicine with "the danger for scientific overkill of general practice" (1998: 187). He argued against further expansion of Evidence-Based Medicine into clinical practice by claiming a unique rationality for general practice gained by personal experience and expressed in "the art of improvisation and individualization" (ibid.: 188). He described the ideal physician by referring to Aristotle as characterized by "personalized competence, an amalgam of knowledge, instincts, feelings and experience" (ibid.: 187), which might be destroyed by science. In an editorial on the assembly, titled "Evidence Based Medicine – Part or End of the Art in Medicine?", a physician expressed his reluctance against Evidence-Based Medicine while ironically acknowledging in phrases adopted from the language of Evidence-Based Medicine: "Sure, it is only a feeling, some experience – located at the bottom end of evidence – gained in 15 years of working in practice that explains my continuous reservation. Critically evaluated, it might hide mere intellectual laziness or pure inability" (Altorfer 1997: 561).

Reluctance toward Evidence-Based Medicine is commonly described through the non-congruence of clinical science producing numerical data from large populations and the work of the practitioner being directed at the individual patient and

---

supporting key conclusions with only a subset of relevant references, has been shown to be both non-reproducible and, as a scientific exercise, of low mean scientific quality" (1997: 13).

his/her specific situation, the art of medicine. In the words of the general practitioner Markus Mader:

> "I think this Evidence-Based Medicine abstracts in a certain sense from individual destiny, and that cannot always be allowed. It is a general statement for a general population, but not for the individual. And I would always like to let the individual decision depend also on other factors than the ones known to be useful."

In concluding the interview, Markus Mader believed that his very insistence on "other factors than the ones known to be useful" are crucial to allow for a continuous care relation with his patient:

> "As soon as I don't respect her territory anymore and start to make demands: okay, now listen![135] Here, new paper: treatment recommendations! If I fully identify with that, it will become very difficult." (Markus Mader)

The statements express an insistence on individual decision-making against following Evidence-Based Medicine's "general statement over a general population". In supporting "Total Quality Management", an alternative pathway toward improving medical care in general practice, Markus Mader was active in setting new standards in family practice. He described Total Quality Management with the aim "that everybody who participates in a process is involved in the improvement of this process"[136]. Markus Mader's efforts for improving the work of the general practitioner through introducing new methods underlines that the reluctance toward Evidence-Based Medicine amongst general practitioners cannot merely be discredited as ignorance or a stubborn resistance to change.

Evidence-Based Medicine emphasizes the ambiguity in the role of the physician in contemporary medicine. On the one hand, medical work is defined through the interaction with the individual patient where treatment is negotiated based upon anamnesis and diagnosis. This definition of medical work stresses the individual skills of the physician and the adaptation of medical knowledge to the patient and his/her unique situation. The focus is on the "other factors than the ones known to be useful" mentioned above by Markus Mader, on variety as opposed to standardization. On the other hand, physicians are increasingly seen as mediators between medical science and the patient. They may fear their role to be reduced to the mere implementation of recommendations generated from the results of clinical research, a process often referred to as transforming medical work into "cook-book medicine"

---

[135] He hits his fist on the table.

[136] Total Quality Management is a concept taken over from business management where it received a lot of attention in the 1990s. The concept assumes that "the worker is a partner with management in a continuously changing process of making quality products that fit customers' continuously changing needs" (Martin 1996a: 154). It sets the ideal of corporate bodies as lean, flexible, fast, and adaptive. According to Martin, these ideals correspond to the image of the ideal human body as developed and described by immunology.

(the cook-book being the standards and guidelines). The term stands for physicians' fear that the "art" of medicine loses terrain against "science" to an extent that physicians not only lose their autonomy and freedom of decision (Conroy and Shannon 1995), but that also a major part of their skills becomes obsolete to a point that their work is reduced to slavishly following the cook-book recipes written up by experts. The following figure tries to illustrate these conflicts resulting for the physician from the expanding influence of clinical science on medical practice: the skills of the physician in the individual diagnostic and therapeutic process and the interaction with the patient lose importance with the increasing demand to shape and standardize these processes according to the findings of research and to the recommendations written down in guidelines. The physician fears his/her role to be reduced to the mere implementation of research and guidelines.

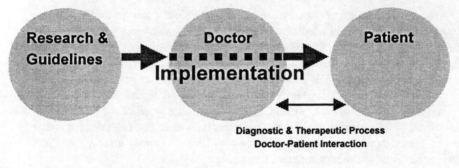

*Figure 14. "Science" expanding into medical work*

Confronted with resistance against Evidence-Based Medicine on the grounds outlined above, Sackett and colleagues perform a balancing act in their dedicated argumentation for their approach. While they are never tire of citing evidence for the inadequacy of decision-making in medical practice, they assure physicians that their art remains central when practicing Evidence-Based Medicine (or, as they shortly and affectionately name it, "EBM"): "However, before we go any further, we want to stress that EBM builds on and reinforces, but never replaces, clinical skills, clinical judgment and clinical experience. If you want to practice EBM, merge it with becoming the best history taker and clinical examiner you can be, incorporate it into becoming the most thoughtful diagnostician and therapist you can become and consolidate it in your evolution into an effective, efficient, caring and compassionate clinician" (Sackett et al. 1997: 5).

The "cook-book" argument against Evidence-Based Medicine is similarly countered by stressing that the integration of evidence into practice means combining it with expertise and adapting it to the patient's view: "Evidence-based medicine is not 'cook-book' medicine. Because it requires a bottom-up approach that integrates the best external evidence with individual clinical expertise and patient choice, it cannot result in slavish, cook-book approaches to individual patient care. External evidence can inform, but can never replace, individual clinical expertise that decides whether the external evidence applies to the individual patient at all and, if so, how it should be integrated into a clinical decision" (Sackett et al. 1997: 3-4). The authors thus use the very key elements usually describing the art of medicine and brought forward against Evidence-Based Medicine – i.e. individual clinical expertise and patient choice – to convince reluctant physicians of Evidence-Based Medicine. A Swiss adherent of Evidence-Based Medicine argued similarly by describing Evidence-Based Medicine as supporting the art of medicine: "Some people maintain that EBM is cook-book medicine. That is not correct. What we call the art of medicine can be practiced better when using EBM" (Bucher 1997: 596).

## 6.4. THE VOICE OF EXPERIENCE

The struggle between the science and art of medical practice is a struggle over which type of medical knowledge is central to medical practice. Knowledge is distinguished into personal experience on the one hand and scientific findings on the other. The internist "Barry Siegler", as portrayed by Hahn, expresses the tensions between these two types of knowledge: "He is extremely skeptical about findings in the literature. He says, 'The stuff you read in the literature, 90 percent is bullshit, maybe 97 percent, maybe even 98 percent.... You can quote me.' As with laboratory results, Barry uses statistical studies to confirm what he already believes. The standing knowledge by which he works significantly shapes the knowledge he may come by" (1995: 194). Barry Siegler's quote indicates his distrust of medical science and his reluctance to incorporate scientific findings into his practice. According to Hahn, such incorporation only takes place when these findings support Siegler's practice and they thus only have a limited potential to modify it. Amongst the general practitioners we interviewed, scientific findings also were discussed in opposition to personal experience. Although citing evidence from "studies" was often used as symbolic capital, personal experience with individual patients tended to be constructed as frequently clashing with statistical evidence and to be given more weight in case of conflict. François Neher for example compared his patient interviewed by us with another of his HIV patients who also has a favorable course of HIV:

> "Funnily enough I just realized that the other non-progressor is also such a character. HIV is really no subject for him, he speaks about Harley Davidson motorcycles and smoking pot or about going to America and things like that, which are much more interesting to him than HIV. Well, you could say...– of course, that's based on my experience, after all it is not statistically relevant – but it is remarkable that it might be a good idea not to think all day long about HIV in order to remain a non-progressor."

Based upon two patients in his practice, François Neher hypothesized on a possible association between attitude and non-progression of HIV. He knew that such a hypothesis is beyond statistical relevance, but the liveliness of the personal experience with these two patients made the idea to some degree more convincing than a statistical finding read in a study, expressed through an impersonal p-value. Acknowledging that the idea is "based on my experience, after all it is not statistically relevant", he was aware of the tensions between personal experience and scientific findings and of the fact that speaking of experience was increasingly suspicious[137], and he knew that his conclusion therefore might be interpreted as naïve.

When talking about his view of the new triple therapies, another physician interviewed expressed his doubts about their overall impact, yet he acknowledged that they seemed to be useful when a person progressed towards AIDS. Lacking personal experience with treatment in his own practice, he did not cite statistical evidence (which he probably was confronted with through reading and attending further education) in order to underline the therapies' effectiveness against AIDS and death, but recounted the experience told by a colleague caring for a large number of HIV patients in his practice. Thus, even in the absence of personal experience, a colleague's experience still seems more convincing than the results of clinical studies:

> "He has some 50 to 80 HIV patients in his practice, and he said that before these therapies, he had about one to two deaths per month, and now since, say, April last year until the end of the year none." (Jonas Ender)

Developing his ideas on the concept of voices taken from Mishler (1984), Atkinson (1995) showed that medical discourse does not articulate a single lifeworld. Instead, the production and reproduction of medical knowledge draws from alternating frames of reference, ranging from personal knowledge expressed in biographically grounded narratives to the de-contextualized and impersonal knowledge of clinical science. Physicians thus speak both with the voices of experience and of science, and these voices also express different, often competing modes of claiming authority. The senior physician for example is allowed and bound to speak with the voice of experience to a junior physician. Through the senior's prolonged medical experience, s/he will almost automatically be in the privileged position vis-à-vis a junior when speaking with the voice of experience. While knowledge thus grows over time and with seniority in the experience-model, the very opposite tends to happen in the evidence-model of medical knowledge. Sackett et al. cited studies showing that acquiring knowledge in practice through the traditional methods of reading journals (not enough) and asking colleagues (who did not read enough, either) was associated with a deterioration of knowledge and performance with time (Sackett et al. 1997).

---

[137] See DelVecchio Good (1995a) cited below.

Adherents of Evidence-Based Medicine indeed describe their approach as a means of overcoming traditional hierarchies in medicine. Status formerly linked through seniority to the biography of the physician is replaced by the skills to gain access to the relevant types of information: "Finally, authoritarian clinicians may see evidence based medicine as a threat. It may cause them to lose face by sometimes exposing their current practice as obsolete or occasionally even dangerous. At times it will alter the dynamics of the team, removing hierarchical distinctions that are based on seniority; some will rue the day when a junior member of the team, by conducting a search and critical appraisal, has as much authority and respect as the team's most senior member" (Rosenberg and Donald 1995: 1125). While developing and advocating new types of knowledge, new skills of acquiring it[138] and new channels for its diffusion, the adherents of Evidence-Based Medicine demonstrate awareness for the fact that these changes entail new power relations. They are longing with almost revolutionary spirit for the day "some will rue" when traditional hierarchies are evened out because junior physicians traditionally lower in the hierarchy overcome their subordination by gaining access to knowledge through new channels not linked to traditional hierarchies. Such predictions certainly contain a strategic element of agitation[139]. By addressing junior physicians as their agents of change the adherents of Evidence-Based Medicine seem to take strategic advantage of what Bourdieu (1993) described as a common feature of any social field, i.e. the struggle between the newcomers and the long-established members of the field. Whoever holds authority within a field tends to defend orthodox values while the newcomers still lacking authority are more likely to seek revolutionary change in order to improve their own position within the field. In this sense, junior physicians are indeed the most likely to adhere to the new methods of Evidence-Based Medicine in order to gain authority in the field of medicine.

While until recently it remained unproblematic for physicians to combine different types of knowledge, including experience and evidence, it became increasingly suspicious with the developments of the last decade. "The common refrain in medicine – 'in my experience...' – has come to be viewed with skepticism, especially since the rise of clinical epidemiology" (DelVecchio Good 1995a: 54-55). Evidence-Based Medicine opened the way for various approaches which attempt to formalize decision-making in clinical practice and to overcome the broadly discussed problem that the physician is implicitly or explicitly basing his/her decisions

---

[138] Among the central skills demanded from the new physician is a profound knowledge in statistics to interpret the probabilities and p-values symbolizing the scientific bases of his/her practice (Le Pen 1999).

[139] Explicit awareness of the exponents of Evidence-Based Medicine for the changing intra-professional power relations stands in contrast to their silence around extra-professional economic and political power entering medicine partly through instruments such as guidelines belonging to the domain of Evidence-Based Medicine (see chapters 6.7. and 6.8.).

on the limited personal experience with individual patients (Speich 1997). Both individual cases and personal experience are, as also expressed by the physicians cited above, more vivid and concrete than numeric probabilities read in journal articles and thus tend to be overvalued in decision-making. A growing body of research on physicians' decision-making is developed with the implicit or explicit aim of challenging "nonscientific drug prescribing" (Schwartz et al. 1989: 577) and changing the fact that despite knowing standards and guidelines "GPs often do not comply with these scientifically-based standards" (Veldhuis et al. 1998: 1833). This finding resembles insight from research in health behavior: knowledge per se does not necessarily translate into behavior. Or, when translating into behavior, it might not be the behavior that health professionals find desirable and reasonable. As the example of physicians' "compliance" with guidelines shows, however, health professionals themselves do not necessarily behave according to the logic and reason of researchers and policy makers. If physicians' behavior thus becomes analyzed in a way similar to their patients' behavior, similar mechanisms are likely to be found.

Analyzing physicians' decision-making is not limited to distinguishing between personal experience and clinical science as the basis for decisions. Whereas some researchers are trying to convince physicians to integrate data from clinical trials into their decision-making, others are already looking further by evaluating how this scientific data consulted by physicians is translated into clinical decisions. A number of studies have shown that decisions vary greatly according to the type of numbers given when reporting study results (Bobbio et al. 1994; Bucher et al. 1994; Forrow et al. 1992; Naylor et al. 1992). These studies have shown that physicians are more willing to prescribe drugs when reading the relative risk reduction achieved through a treatment, which is commonly used in trial reports and drug advertisement, than when reading the absolute risk reduction. Relative risk reduction tends to give higher percentages than absolute risk reduction especially when the patients' susceptibility to a disease is low (Sackett and Cook 1994). An example used in one of the cited studies was derived from the Helsinki Heart Study. In this study, patients were treated over five years either with treatment or with a placebo. The outcome of the study can be expressed either in a 1.4% absolute reduction or in a 34% relative reduction of cardiac events or deaths through treatment (Bobbio et al. 1994). These two percentages result from the same clinical trial and thus express the same outcome, though with a different type of calculation. Most of us have problems understanding the mathematical difference in calculating relative and absolute risk, and we tend to be more impressed by a 34% relative risk reduction than by a 1.4% absolute risk reduction, regardless of how it is calculated. It therefore seems of little surprise that the higher percentages expressing relative risk reduction make physicians more willing to prescribe treatment. And it seems just as intelligible that drug companies prefer their study results to be described by the relative risk reduction. The different types of calculation translate into different sales figures, thus illustrating how the evidence that medicine should be based upon is also subject to strategy and particular interests. As Kaufert pointed out, medical facts take on a form of independent life once they are produced and diffused, an independence partly allowed by the fact that "the main consumers of medical knowledge, the practicing clinicians, are too often methodologically naïve" (1988: 332).

The above cited studies are part of a broad attempt to base medical decision-making on probabilistic thinking, which replaces the mechanistic search for clear answers through the indication of the probability of an outcome. Probabilistic thinking stands for the acknowledgement that uncertainty is inherent to decision-making: "From the vantage point of the probabilistic paradigm, uncertainty is not a residual problem, nor a symptom of failure. It is recognized as a pervasive feature of all decisions and actions" (Atkinson 1995: 112). Thinking in terms of probabilities, calculating and monitoring risk and chance, in turn reflect a fundamental feature of modern societies. If modernity is described as a risk culture, this does not mean that social life has become more risky than it used to be, but that the concept of risk becomes fundamental to the way both lay actors and specialists organize the world (Giddens 1991). According to Fox (1980), medicine is an epicenter in which risk and uncertainty are negotiated. Fox found in her research that the increasing mastery of the probability-reasoning logic is a mechanism for physicians to cope with the uncertainties of their work. Yet replacing clear suggestions for or against a therapy or procedure by the indication of the probability that it will be successful is also bound to increase physicians' uncertainty. Uncertainty increased by probabilistic reasoning may in practice provide yet a further argument against using scientific data. As the family practitioner Goldstein wrote: "With uncertainty all around me, I sometimes long for the security that science appears to offer. Unfortunately, science can no longer offer the comfort that I need. Positivism has long since given way to probability" (1990: 28).

Not only probabilistic reasoning, but already the discussions around which types of knowledge are legitimate and relevant in general practice cause profound uncertainty amongst some physicians. Marco Deville's reflections on the value of individual cases show the dilemma of choosing the "correct" types of evidence under the current pressure on using population-based data from clinical studies as opposed to the individual case study:

> "There is of course nothing but statistics. But anecdotal cases are interesting. Scientifically, an individual case is not interesting, but when you read somewhere in *Focus* or *Facts*[140] or somewhere an individual case about an American who achieved this or that with this combination or that – an individual case, anecdotal – that's also scientifically interesting. You tend to generalize, but sometimes individual cases are firstly interest-

---

[140] Two popular magazines in German speaking countries.

ing and secondly I believe that in these areas you can also evaluate them. Of course, you need statistics, so and so many infected, this therapy and that used, and so forth. But an individual case sometimes is...– well, it does not really belong in the bulletin, but (...) it is more vivid. An individual case is being reported in which someone with a triple combination, with a bomb (...) practically gets a viral load of zero. Many cases are known. That's interesting." (Marco Deville)

Marco Deville's insistence on the value of the individual case is not as deviant as he seems to fear when talking with my colleague who probably represents through his affiliation with a university hospital the scientific pole of medicine. Case studies on individual patients are a common genre in medical journals and in medical education. Social studies give detailed accounts on how medical knowledge is constructed from diverse sources, ranging from case studies to clinical trials (Hunt and Mattingly 1998: 270; Kaufert 1988; Mattingly 1998). The preference of the individual physician for one or the other side of the spectrum can be described through his/her temporal and institutional distance towards medical science and academe. Temporal distance is mainly expressed – as outlined above – in the time elapsed since medical education and the resulting seniority of the physician. Institutional distance is mainly characterized by the boundary between general vs. specialized medicine and physicians with private practice vs. physician-scientists at university clinics. The latter are not only exposed to basic science through researchers invited for lectures, but they themselves practice scientific research, often at the expense of their already scarce free time. In addition, they participate in generating the data for clinical trials often paid by pharmaceutical companies introducing new medication. It thus seems intelligible that they may be less reluctant against scientific evidence and may have better access to it[141] than the average general practitioner.

---

[141] Which certainly does not mean that these doctor-scientists implement scientific evidence in a coherent and straightforward manner. HIV specialists for example describe different treatment "cultures" within the different HIV centers in Switzerland. There are centers known as "treatment hard-liners", others as being reluctant toward treating, and still others are positioned "somewhere in between".

## 6.5. THE MEDIUM IS THE MESSAGE

The demand to base medical practice on medical science partly gained ground through technical innovations providing new means to accessing scientific data. With the availability of personal computers, electronic databases and the Internet, it became at least theoretically possible for any general practitioner to directly access and process vast up-to-date bodies of scientific data[142]. Traditional methods to access information, including traditional types of further education or the consultation of experts, are increasingly discredited for not providing the right answers to a given question (Davis et al. 1995). Valid and useful data are epitomized by the randomized controlled trial which Evidence-Based Medicine is advocating. Finding these data and evaluating them through systematic reviews and meta-analyses[143] may, even for physicians trained and experienced in the approach, require considerable time. Evidence-Based Medicine therefore developed shortcuts to obtain relevant data by preparing systematic reviews and meta-analyses on given subjects and thus taking over part of the workload of data collection and evaluation. The most important media publishing such systematic reviews and meta-analyses include the *Cochrane Library* and the journals *ACP Journal Club* and *Evidence-Based Medicine*, all of them products of the 1990s.

The *Cochrane Library* is published on CD ROM by the Cochrane Collaboration. The organization is named after the British epidemiologist Archie Cochrane who already in the 1970s (Cochrane 1972) drew "attention to our great collective ignorance about the effects of health care. He recognized that people who want to make more informed decisions about health care do not have ready access to reliable reviews of the available evidence"[144]. The Cochrane Centre in Oxford was established in 1992 (Chalmers et al. 1992), and the Cochrane Collaboration, which subsequently published the *Cochrane Library* was founded in 1993 at the initiative of the Centre. In 1998, a new Collaborative Review Group on HIV/AIDS was formed to prepare and collect systematic reviews and meta-analyses on the subject (Rutherford 1998).

---

[142] The importance of these new instruments and techniques leads us back to an insight already gained for the production of scientific facts (chapter 2.3.): the development of specific complexes of instruments and the skills required to utilize them are among the preconditions to reshape knowledge (Rouse 1992).

[143] The meta-analysis is considered to be the most systematic and accurate overview on research on a given problem. It provides a synthesis of given trials which is performed by using specific sorts of statistics (Sackett et al. 1997; Thacker 1988).

[144] As cited from the homepage of the Cochrane Collaboration (March 2, 2000): http://som.flinders.edu.au/fusa/cochrane/cochrane/cc-broch.htm

The *ACP Journal Club* was founded in 1991 by the American College of Physicians ACP. The authors select articles on a given subject according to the methods used in the studies, rewrite them based on their own standards in a shortened one-page version, and ask an expert to write a comment on them. The journal *Evidence Based Medicine* was founded in 1995 again by the ACP in collaboration with the British Medical Journal Publishing Group. It includes work published in the *ACP Journal Club*, systematic reviews from the *Cochrane Library*, and its own review articles. The publishers believe that "*ACP Journal Club* and *Evidence-Based Medicine* will publish the gold that intellectually intense processes will mine from the ore of about 100 of the world's top journals. Doctors owe it to themselves and their patients to make sure that they keep up with what is new and important" (Davidoff et al. 1995: 1086).

An even more direct transformation of research results into instructions for clinical practice than provided by systematic reviews and meta-analyses are clinical guidelines, described as "the distillation of a large body of knowledge into a convenient, readily usable format" (Ellrodt et al. 1997: 1689). Guidelines in the general sense are not a product of Evidence-Based Medicine, but they are much older. According to Eddy, they have been used for centuries to summarize standard and accepted practice. Instead of trying to change those practices, they rather reflect them: "Thus, by the traditional approach, practice policies are not 'designed'. Rather, they evolve, continuously tracking practices in common use" (1990c: 1265). Woolf defined practice guidelines as "the official statements and policies of major organizations and agencies on the proper indications for performing a procedure or treatment or the proper management for specific clinical problems" (1990: 1812)[145]. He held that even in this definition, practice guidelines had been used for more than 50 years. More recent though is the introduction of new approaches to develop guidelines according to the standards of Evidence-Based Medicine. It is through these approaches that guidelines become part of the tools of Evidence-Based Medicine.

The various approaches to develop guidelines once more reflect the tension between "scientific evidence and expert opinion" (Woolf 1992: 950), which is omnipresent in the discourse on medical practice. Traditional approaches are based on consensus development amongst experts who may cite scientific evidence yet without a methodological approach (Woolf 1992). Evidence-based approaches contrast these traditional approaches through their methodology. Eddy (1990b; 1990c) distinguished three different, increasingly sophisticated approaches to developing evidence-based guidelines: Firstly, the "evidence-based approach" explicitly describes the evidence and ties its policy to it. Secondly, the "outcomes-based

---

[145] The article is part of a series on the development, methods, and impact of practice guidelines (Woolf 1990; 1992; 1993).

approach" additionally estimates the outcomes of alternative practices to those rec-ommended. This may be done either through experts' subjective estimation, a method which is obviously not evidence-based, or through formal quantitative tech-niques[146]. Thirdly, the "preference-based approach" complements the outcomes-based approach, performed by using formal quantitative techniques, with the formal assessment of patients' preferences. In this approach, experts' subjective judgment is supposed to be eliminated from the development of guidelines while patients' sub-jective preferences, based on a formal evaluation, become included. That such an approach may be, due to lack of evidence, unrealistic in the case of many interven-tions was also acknowledged by Eddy (1990c). As of 1990, he only knew of prefer-ence-based approaches developed in research programs, and they were rare. Eddy was aware that different actors might react in different ways to this fact: "People who hope for a long list of rigid criteria that can be used in quality-assurance and cost-control programs will be disappointed. People who fear losing their freedom to make decisions will be pleasantly surprised" (1990a: 3084). He proposed that the doctor-patient interaction (and thus, the art of medicine) should compensate for this lack of evidence and scientific certainty: "It is difficult and time-consuming to dis-cuss outcomes and preferences with patients. On the other hand, there is a strong tradition of individual decision making, and most practitioners bridle at the notion of being mere technologists who follow preformed rules. For better or for worse, we have no choice about how much flexibility practitioners should have. The plain fact is that uncertainty, variability of outcomes, and variability of preferences exist, and practice policies must be responsive to those realities"[147] (ibid.).

Our data indicate that guidelines are indeed a major source of information for physicians. This stands in contrast to the still marginal use of the Internet and elec-tronic databases, media which are central if a physician wants to perform systematic reviews and meta-analyses him-/herself.

---

[146] This work is now partly taken over by the meta-analyses published in the journals and databases described above.

[147] The argument in favor of negotiating decisions in the doctor-patient interaction in the face of scien-tific uncertainty resembles the statement by François Neher in chapter 4.4.. He similarly argued in favor of patient preferences in the face of limited knowledge on antiretroviral treatment.

*Table 20. General practitioners' sources of information*

|                                                    | n    | %     |
|----------------------------------------------------|------|-------|
| Bulletin of the Swiss Federal Office of Public Health | 458  | 85.9  |
| Journals, books                                    | 372  | 69.8  |
| HIV center                                         | 247  | 46.3  |
| Other GPs                                          | 196  | 36.8  |
| Conferences                                        | 179  | 33.6  |
| Further education at HIV center                    | 113  | 21.2  |
| Internet                                           | 37   | 6.9   |
| Databases                                          | 31   | 5.8   |
| Other complementary therapists                     | 21   | 3.9   |
| Other sources                                      | 25   | 4.7   |
| Total                                              | 533  | 100.0 |

As table 20 shows, the Internet (6.9%) and electronic databases (5.8%) were used only by a small minority of general practitioners as sources of information on HIV. Since using these media is a precondition to performing systematic reviews and meta-analyses, it may be assumed that the average Swiss general practitioners is far from the ideals envisioned by the advocates of Evidence-Based Medicine. On the other hand, the bulletin of the Swiss Federal Office of Public Health where treatment guidelines are published was consulted by a majority (85.9%) of the general practitioners. Reading articles or consulting books on HIV/AIDS was also frequent (69.8%), followed by receiving information from the HIV center (46.3%) usually obtained through collaboration in the care of individual patients. One third (36.8%) of the general practitioners received information through exchange with other general practitioners while exchange across disciplinary boundaries with complementary therapists remained rare (3.9%). Formal education, including conferences (33.6%) and further education provided by the HIV centers (21.2%) reached a minority, though of considerable extent, of general practitioners[148]. The number of different sources of information consulted was associated with the practical relevance of HIV/AIDS: general practitioners who cared for HIV/AIDS patients consulted a higher number of sources[149] than their colleagues without HIV/AIDS patients (p<0.001). Amongst the general practitioners caring for HIV/AIDS patients, those with a higher number of patients (>2 patients) consulted more sources of

---

[148] According to a systematic review of the effect of continuing medical education strategies (Davis et al. 1995), formal medical education activities like conferences had little impact on physicians' performance and/or on patients' health care outcomes. The authors of the review concluded that the less effective strategies in continuing medical education seem to be amongst the ones most commonly used.

[149] The number of sources consulted by a physician was dichotomized (0-3 sources vs. >3 sources) in order to calculate the association.

information (p=0.012)[150]. This data highlights that information-seeking in the general practice is guided by the need for information in patient care. The more a physician is confronted with HIV/AIDS patients in his practice, the more sources of information he consults. Furthermore, general practitioners seem to select the sources according to their skills in accessing and handling the medium and according to the time required to gain the desired information. Treatment recommendations are short and – although also available on the Internet – easily accessible in the traditional form of a widely distributed journal. In contrast, consulting electronic databases and the Internet requires the use of computers, and performing systematic reviews or meta-analyses demands specialized methodological and statistical knowledge, and it may be time-consuming. These new media and methods are therefore of marginal use in general practice.

Luca Granges whose narrative introduces this chapter is convinced that the electronic media will revolutionize medicine by empowering patients through access to information:

> "I am personally convinced that the electronic media and also the systematic appraisal of information, as it is for example done by the *Cochrane Collaboration*, will in the wider context of medicine, not only in the field of HIV, revolutionize medicine. People that want it will finally become informed consumers. It will provide the possibilities that people can inform themselves and make free choices between different physicians. They will learn to judge the quality of clinics or practicing physicians, or, as it will probably be the case in the United States, of collaborating groups of physicians. I think such a judgment is urgently required. I prefer the informed consumer over the non-informed one. Of course, he is less pleasant and more demanding, but actually I prefer that, especially in the case of situations as complex as in HIV."

Luca Granges creates a vision of the informed consumer through electronic access to information. Measured by his standards, most general practitioners in our sample would have to be declared as "non-informed" consumers of medical knowledge, considering that they have only marginally taken part in the electronic revolution. Should Luca Granges' vision really become true, the patients might soon move ahead of their doctors.

General practitioners' tendency toward traditional methods of information-seeking was also apparent during our interviews. When talking about treatment decisions, they usually had a copy of the Swiss treatment guidelines (not always the latest edition) from the bulletin of the Swiss Federal Office of Public Health readily at hand. The physicians more involved or interested in HIV care recounted what they had heard in further education or from their colleagues, in some cases even in formal exchange rounds on HIV/AIDS amongst colleagues. While some physicians also read journal articles on HIV/AIDS, they did not conduct their own literature

---

[150] Tables not shown.

searches on the computer – in fact, the computer tended to be located in the entrance room on the receptionist's desk. The following quote where a general practitioner told how he was looking for information when his patient was confronted with the decision whether or not to start treatment outlines the information-seeking process of a rather committed physician:

> "I must say, back then I informed myself a bit, mostly with these official statements of the Federal Office of Public Health (...). These guidelines from a year ago have been withdrawn now, but I have actually already heard in further education that also at the HIV centers nobody complied with them anymore. Well, the Federal Office of Public Health lags behind, unfortunately, I must say. (...[151]). That's about what I get out of further education or discussions – I have some colleagues, I know a bit those practitioners in town that are very active in treating HIV patients, I do not belong to them, but I know some of them, some have quite high numbers {of HIV patients}. And from them I got some information and discussed some things.
>
> ck: And you also said that you participated in further education?
>
> Yes, the last major thing was half a day on HIV therapies at the university hospital. (...).
>
> ck: Do you as a general practitioner feel sufficiently informed?
>
> In those further education activities they said – that was new to me – that we could forget this cross scheme with so and so much CD4 and so and so much viral load. Somebody, I don't remember who it was, said: the real indication for treatment is that the patient wants to be treated. Period. For the moment at least that is about what they tell you. If you can say it stood the test of time... Everything is continuously changing so much. In that sense, I also think a bit: well, after all they are no better than anybody else. They tell you something and two years later they tell you something different. I mean, they also make their mistakes, but their mistakes are so to speak somehow officially sanctioned mistakes. But after all you know little. That also takes some pressure from me." (Jonas Ender)

Jonas Ender described how he informed himself through official guidelines (which he distrusted to some degree since they "lag behind" scientific developments), through further education at the HIV clinic and through colleagues in town he had formal and informal exchanges with. The criticism that the official guidelines lag behind the scientific development reflects the most commonly cited reason for not adhering to guidelines as given by Australian general practitioners with a high caseload of HIV patients and ongoing medical education in HIV/AIDS: These general practitioners argued that they did not adhere to the guidelines because they found them to be out of date (Smith et al. 2000). Jonas Ender's plot of the information-seeking process is related to this criticism: given that knowledge transmitted by the experts is continuously changing and thus becoming outdated, he feels that also experts make their "officially sanctioned mistakes", a feeling that takes some pressure from his own decisions. He thus perceives the uncertainty of medical knowledge not only as a burden. Rather, it may also turn into the strategic advantage of

---

[151] He recounts his version of the current knowledge on HIV treatment.

the practicing physician by allowing more freedom in decision-making, a line of reasoning which is further reflected in the following chapter.

## 6.6. STATE-OF-THE-ART IGNORANCE

Uncertainty has become a fashionable topic in medicine. Basic to the development of the subject is the research conducted over several decades by Renée Fox (1980), a medical sociologist. In her first work on uncertainty, Fox distinguished from her empirical research three different types of uncertainty: Firstly, uncertainty resulting from incomplete or imperfect mastery of available knowledge, secondly, uncertainty resulting from limitations in current medical knowledge, and thirdly, uncertainty resulting from the difficulties in distinguishing between the first two types, i. e. between personal ignorance and the limitations of current medical knowledge (Fox 1957).

As our research was conducted during a major paradigm change in HIV, uncertainty became for patients and their physicians a main feature in the decision-making process. While new studies from basic and clinical science were published and new antiretroviral drugs were brought to trials and quickly became approved, HIV and its treatment were constantly redefined. The HIV specialist Luca Granges tried to describe the uncertainty in patient care that resulted from these rapid changes:

> "Well, I simply try to counsel people to the best of my knowledge and belief, and that changes constantly. As you know, in the last 15, 16 months really major developments have been achieved and new drugs came, and the guidelines are turned upside down every six months. Well, maybe not turned upside down, but completed. (...). I try to give my patients recommendations to the best of my knowledge and belief and according the state-of-the-art knowledge or ignorance, and I also try to check if these guidelines or what is currently considered to be optimal treatment, suit the patient."

Luca Granges, who himself was competent in the field of Evidence-Based Medicine, rephrased his initial description of the guidelines as being "turned upside down" to being "completed" every six months. Nevertheless, given the rapid changes, he wondered if the "state-of-the art" in HIV practice could be defined as "knowledge" or rather represented "ignorance". Thus he could also not only rely on his "knowledge" when counseling patients, but also on his "belief". What is expressed in this knowledge/ignorance and knowledge/belief opposition is the fundamental uncertainty resulting, according to Fox' typology, from limitations in current medical knowledge and from difficulties in distinguishing between the limitations of current knowledge and personal ignorance. Remarkably, this uncertainty seems to become more pronounced with the rapid expansion of knowledge than through the limitations per se (Fox 1980). In the context of the limitation of knowledge remaining rather stable, an agreement is reached on what can and cannot be done. In contrast, the rapid expansion of knowledge firstly increases the awareness that decisions taken recently have already become outdated and thus "false" from the new point of view. Secondly, it makes clear that decisions taken at present might just as quickly become false with future developments. The rapid expansion and revision of knowledge blurs the boundary between knowledge and belief or ignorance. Franz Jann described how this situation increases both the physician's and the patient's uncertainty:

> "When I sometimes look through medical histories and see what I wrote half a year ago, I think it can't be true that I wrote that. And the very same also happens to any patient coming to us every six months and getting totally different information than the last time he came."

While ever-changing recommendations given by the physician may diminish the patient's confidence and increase his/her uncertainty, the same applies to the physician in relation to constantly revised expert knowledge and treatment recommendations. Jonas Ender cited in the above chapter spoke in this context of experts' "officially sanctioned mistakes", thus of the fact that also official statements may inevitably prove wrong within a short time. François Neher described the treatment guidelines as representing "again and again current state-of-the-art ignorance", thus using the same phrase as Luca Granges cited above. Although I was less concerned with treatment than physicians or people with HIV/AIDS, I was also often puzzled by the changing attitudes and recommendations of the physicians I worked with. As soon as I started believing that it might be a good idea for a person with HIV to take antiretroviral treatment as early as possible, the same physicians that had advocated this idea had already started countering it by arguing the development of treatment resistance and the problems of long-term adherence. My confusion though was less troubling than it probably is for a physician as I did not have patients who counted on my recommendation for their decision, and it was especially less troubling than for a person with HIV/AIDS whose life may depend on treatment.

Uncertainty though does not only limit, but also liberate medical work. The ambivalence towards uncertainty expressed in the above chapter by Jonas Ender runs throughout medical interpretations of the subject. Uncertainty is given positive meaning mainly in two interrelated contexts. Firstly, it helps physicians to underpin the importance of their professional competence in the face of limited scientific evidence. DelVecchio Good showed how oncologists define their competence through the very fact that treatment technologies and scientific uncertainties are constantly evolving. In the perspective of the oncologists, their competence arises from using routine technologies in new ways "and from uncertainties about the efficacy of treatments and of the biomedical sciences that underpin the clinical craft" (1995a: 4).

Naylor, a representative of Evidence-Based Medicine, supported this role of professional competence, or the art of medicine, as a compensation for scientific uncertainty in medicine which "seems to consist of a few things we know, a few things we think we know (but probably don't), and lots of things we don't know at all" (1995: 840). He argued that there are a number of reasons why uncertainty will remain despite clinical science, a fact that also guideline writers should rather acknowledge than hide. A Canadian compendium on preventive health care served in his description as a positive example for such an acknowledgement since it characterized a large number of procedures as not supported by scientific evidence: "There are no less than seventy-six manoeuvres characterised by inconclusive evidence and labelled as 'grade C recommendations', where decision-making must be guided by factors other than medical scientific evidence" (ibid.: 841). According to Naylor, these factors include clinical reasoning based on experience, analogy, and extrapolation as well as communicating with the patient to elicit and respect his/her preferences and to help him/her live with uncertainty: "More generally, the prudent application of evaluative sciences will affirm rather than obviate the need for the art of medicine" (ibid.: 841). The art of medicine is thus mainly acknowledged as a inevitable compensation for the "Grey Zones of Clinical Practice", as Naylor titled his article, which resist standardization through clear recommendations and thus produce uncertainty. Yet ultimately this art is qualified as the less desirable aspect of medical work. As Naylor closed his article: "let us agree that good clinical practice will always blend the art of uncertainty with the science of probability. But let us also hope that the blend can be weighted heavily towards science, whenever and wherever sound evidence is brought to light" (ibid.: 841-842).

A second context in which uncertainty is attributed positive meaning is in defense of physicians' individual decision-making against external control and attempts for rationalization of medical practice. The uncertainty inherent to medical work is a major argument against economic, political, and public control of medicine. In an article titled "Guidelines, Enthusiasms, Uncertainty and the Limits to Purchasing", McKee and Clarke for example presented the uncertainty inherent in clinical practice as the main argument against purchasing that is limited to medical services recommended in guidelines[152]: "The most enthusiastic advocates for the purchasing of guidelines and protocols may have paid insufficient attention to the uncertainty inherent in clinical practice, with the imposition of a spurious rationality on sometimes inherently irrational processes" (1995: 101). Patient preferences are among the reasons why medical practice cannot be rationalized and thus has to face the "challenges of balancing the desire for protocol based uniformity with the needs of individual patients" (ibid.).

---

[152] They describe the purchasing of guidelines and protocols as follows: "This vision sees all interventions progressively being evaluated by randomized controlled trials and purchasers undertaking comprehensive assessment of need that will indicate which services should be purchased: locally adapted guidelines will be implemented by all providers; purchasers will buy not activities but guidelines or protocols" (McKee and Clarke 1995: 101.)

In an editorial in the *Lancet*, uncertainty even seemed to emerge as the last line of defense of the physician's authority threatened to be undermined by a variety of non-medical actors. The author gives a rather apocalyptic image of how these actors are claiming control over medical practice based on new sources of information: "An avalanche of more reliable information about medical practice is anticipated in the coming years, with reviews made publicly available in a far more open and critical environment and with scientific commentary written in a style accessible to users of health services. In addition, better hospital statistics are expected to inform managers of local provider performance. This new information is emerging at a time when the mass media no longer keep a respectable distance from the medical profession but display a voracious interest in doctoring. Simultaneously, an army of new types of academic commentator on medicine has arisen – economists, statisticians, sociologists. Consumer groups have been born, some of them wielding considerable power" (Editorial 1995: 1449). The "avalanche" of new types of information produced and spread by different actors may lead to a deterioration of physician authority (and income) through informed patients taking over medical decisions themselves: "The electronic individualists imagine a future in which the patient largely replaces and radically subordinates the physician. Like the eighteenth century aristocrat with an amateur interest in medicine, but this time empowered with proper scientific information from league tables, CD-ROMs, and the Internet, the consumer of the future 'will organise most of his medical needs from his own home…dialling up a doctor or a pharmacist only if the need arises'" (ibid.: 1450)[153]. Similarly as in the article by McKee and Clarke cited above, medical uncertainty is the main argument against this vision of the subordinated physician: "But are these electronic visionaries themselves fully wired? To begin with, reviews concerning common interventions may simply document uncertainty or show the failure of researchers to identify outcomes relevant to service users." The author argues that it is misleading to believe that medical power rests solely on the monopoly of scientific information. S/he therefore concludes, with what seems to be considerable relief, that the access to new sources of information will not diminish medical power: "Thus, more public information, or more sceptical attitudes to what we already know, are unlikely by themselves to impair medical power, for that power seems to rest as much on uncertainty as on technical expertise. Uncertainty in the face of disease and death fosters a compelling need for patients to trust someone – and a reciprocal authority among doctors. A leap of faith will always be needed" (ibid.: 1450-1451). Uncertainty in this argumentation turns into the strategic advantage of the physician struggling for power and authority.

---

[153] The image of this future patient shows similarities with the description of the informed patient given in chapter 6.5. by Luca Granges, with the notable difference that Luca Granges welcomed the idea of an informed patient.

## 6.7. WHO CONTROLS MEDICINE?

In her broad evaluation of the meaning of competence in American medicine, DelVecchio Good placed the efforts launched by the medical profession to guide, evaluate, and review the work of the medical practitioner into the context of an eroding authority and autonomy of the profession. She illustrated the demise of the "golden era of trust" (1995a: 11) with the increase in malpractice claims against physicians in the United States, starting in the 1960s and peaking in the 1980s. Initially, physicians reacted to malpractice suits through a discourse about uncertainty inherent to medical practice and about redesigning the doctor-patient interaction, thus arguing with the "art" of medicine as a cure to the malaise. Only gradually and reluctantly, professional organizations introduced activities to reduce the variability in medical practice by developing written practice standards and clinical guidelines to base medical work on scientific standards[154]. They thus changed their strategy from defending the variability of medical practice as inherent to the "art" of medicine towards seeking standardization based upon scientific research. Although unclear if due to a causal association, malpractice claims did according to Woolf (1992) in the case of anesthesia indeed fall with the introduction of guidelines.

Besides being a reaction to malpractice suits, the introduction of standards and guidelines was also as a consequence of rising health care costs. They provided the background for political actors to call for effectiveness research and for the establishment of criteria to assess the necessity and appropriateness of medical interventions. In intense negotiations between the state and physician associations, standards and guidelines were agreed on as appropriate means to accomplish greater control over medical practice. An alternative suggestion to achieve such control, the establishment of national expenditure targets, was strongly opposed by organized medicine[155] (Woolf 1990).

---

[154] Eddy described the difference between standards and guidelines, which he united under the term "practice policies", through their compulsoriness for the individual physician: "'Guidelines' are intended to be flexible. They serve as reference point, not rigid criteria. Guidelines *should* be followed in *most* cases, but there is an understanding that, depending on the patient, the setting, the circumstances, or other factors, guidelines can and should be tailored to serve individual needs. (...). 'Standards' in contrast, are intended to be inflexible. They define correct practice, and should be followed, not tailored" (1990b: 878, emphases in original). The definition of the two terms and their distinction through the degree of control left to the physician (none in the case of standards) indicates the relevance of these instruments in decreasing physician autonomy.

[155] According to Woolf, the American Medical Association reasoned with patients' well-being against expenditure targets by stating "that expenditure targets could force restrictions on medically necessary services and thereby ration care for elderly and disabled persons" (1990: 1812). In analogy to the current discussions around economic interventions through the state in Switzerland, as outlined below, it may be assumed that the American Medical Association was concerned not only about patients' well-being, but also about its own members' financial well-being.

Thus, both in the legal and the economic arena, medical associations agreed to standards and guidelines in an attempt to preserve professional autonomy against external intervention. With practice guidelines which control medicine through scientific criteria developed within medicine, medical associations could retain some of the power of controlling their work. Yet guidelines came to be viewed by some physicians as a challenge to the autonomy in their practice, creating the paradoxical situation that activities intended to delimit external influence also limited internal autonomy. "Promoting new efforts at professional self-regulation requires a balancing act, one able to disarm doctors' traditional resistance to regulation, defuse protests against encroachment of clinical autonomy, and distance the moral and judgmental dimensions of critiques of customary services" (DelVecchio Good 1995a: 20). Physicians' resistance against these efforts of "'big brotherism'" (ibid.: 21) were countered by organized medicine through the argument that they were preferable to guidelines dictated by insurance companies or the state.

Yet the power that guidelines should retain is increasingly shared with other actors such as the state and insurance companies. In the United States, the power of the state is symbolized by the establishment of the Agency for Health Care Policy and Research AHCPR in 1989: "The establishment of this agency carries important implications to medicine. It places the government in the role of promoting the development and dissemination of practice guidelines on how physicians should evaluate and manage medical conditions" (Woolf 1990: 1813). The paradigmatic image of the economically and politically controlled physician is the employee at the Health Maintenance Organization HMO. Derber (1985) predicted physicians' proletarianization and loss of control through organizationally-based practices as part of a new political economy of medicine. In a similar argumentation, Annas (1995) described the patient as a consumer making decisions in an egalitarian position to his/her physician as a myth since decisions are actually relegated from the physician to corporate entities.

In Switzerland, the economic role of the government and of private insurance companies in medicine is currently negotiated through the restructuring of medical tariffs in the TarMed project. Besides raising polemics around the respective status of general and specialized medicine (see chapter 5.2.), the project provokes efforts of the professional organizations to keep the power to control the economic aspects of medicine within the profession. The project was launched in 1986 by representatives of insurance companies and by the Swiss Medical Association FMH, influenced by scientific data provided from the National Research Project No. 8 ("Economic efficiency and effectiveness in the Swiss health services") of the Swiss National Science Foundation (Brunner 1997a). From the very beginning on, the institutional setting therefore involved the main institutional actors interested in determining medical tariffs: the state, insurance companies, and medical associations.

The role of the state profoundly changed over the long years of negotiating new tariffs. While initially the state provided the scientific basis for the project, it increasingly tried to actively bring the project to a conclusion as medical representatives fighting over tariffs of their respective specialties kept protracting it. With the new health insurance law in Switzerland, the state received the power to set the tariffs if the parties involved do not find an agreement, thus reflecting the decreasing autonomy of the medical profession on the legal level. So far, the Department of the Interior did not take advantage of this possibility. According to the president of the FMH, Hans Heinrich Brunner, state interference is the main problem in the revision of the medical tariffs, involving more conflicts than the resistance of specialists. As Brunner was quoted in a newspaper article on the role of the Department of the Interior in the TarMed negotiations: "'It was as if someone asks to join the meal and when sitting at the table makes more and more outrageous demands', Brunner described the hurt feelings of the FMH" (Sennhauser 2000: 14). In another attack against external interference in tariffs, the FMH answered on its homepage a question of the physician "B.B. in M." who described TarMed as "the monster that Brunner and partners were breeding for years in the dungeons of the FMH" as follows: "What do you believe, dear B.B. in M., what would this 'monster' look like if we hadn't taken part in its breeding – or whether it really would have turned into a monster if we had bred it ourselves? Have fun thinking about it and best regards from Brunner and partners"[156].

## 6.8. EVIDENCE-BASED MEDICINE AS A TROJAN HORSE?

As I have outlined so far in this chapter, Evidence-Based Medicine serves as the medium for and the symbol of profound changes in the organization of medicine. Its founders and advocates declare it as a formalization and dissemination of "evidence", being the relevant type of knowledge. They thus redefine which types of knowledge are legitimate to base decisions in medical practice on, a process that involves an implicit or explicit establishment of new power relations in medicine. Knowledge developed in clinical trials and codified in statistical significance gains importance as opposed to the personal competence and experience of the physician. New institutions and media developed to produce, gather and distribute these forms of knowledge diminish individual expertise. According to the exponents of Evidence-Based Medicine, these developments quasi naturally bring about changes also

---

[156] www.fmh.ch/d/tarmed, January 18, 2000. The language used by physicians among colleagues in a forum as official as the homepage of the FMH might be worth – and maybe fun – thinking about by medical anthropologists and other researchers in social and cultural studies of medicine.

in the power relations between practicing physicians, for example within a team of hospital physicians where seniority based upon work experience and gradual ascendancy in position may lose some of the power linked to it.

Along with these changing intra-professional power relations, the formal codification of knowledge through Evidence-Based Medicine also constitutes and is used as a medium to enhance external surveillance and control of medical practice and physician performance. As outlined in the above chapter, this use for example of guidelines and standards already becomes apparent in the history of these instruments which were agreed on as a compromise to keep away other means of controlling costs and quality of medical care. In fact, policies are established in the United States in order to enforce guidelines. Different states have laws requiring compliance with specific guidelines, and some malpractice insurers mandate compliance as a condition of coverage (Woolf 1993). Woolf aptly noted on the multifaceted interests in medical guidelines represented by different actors: "Although everyone wants practice guidelines to improve the quality of care, only patients care exclusively about clinical outcomes[157]. Clinicians seek improvements in clinical outcomes but also want to limit impositions on autonomy, income, and medical liability. Insurers, employers, public agencies, and other payers want practice guidelines to reduce costs and practice variations. Legislators and politicians want guidelines to decrease public expenditures, and administrators of hospitals and other health care organizations want them to optimize efficiency and risk management. Utilization reviewers want practice guidelines to help identify inappropriate care. Malpractice attorneys want guidelines to help prove negligence" (ibid.: 2647).

The exponents of Evidence-Based Medicine demonstrate considerable awareness for physicians' resistance against interference with their work as long as it is expressed in terms of fearing science to limit the art of medicine, i.e. in terms of intra-medical power relations. In contrast, they remain more silent when it comes to resistance against external economic, political and legal control over medicine through the instruments of Evidence-Based Medicine. Nevertheless, primary care physicians and their representatives, being a main target-group of guidelines, demonstrate awareness for the use of Evidence-Based Medicine – unintended as it might be by its founders – as a means of external control. To use an image of Greek mythology, they seem to fear Evidence-Based Medicine as a Trojan Horse carrying standardization, control, and rationing into medical practice. In an already cited editorial on Evidence-Based Medicine, a general practitioner for example wondered: "Of course the meta-analysis leaves me the freedom of medical decision-making.

---

[157] This is probably true as long as a patient needs medical care. When the same person though leaves her patient role and for example pays her insurance fees, she may also become interested in cutting the costs of medical care.

Nice. But: for how long?" (Altorfer 1997: 561). A primary health care professor warned already in 1992: "Clinical guidelines are rapidly proliferating on both sides of the Atlantic. Mainly intended to improve the quality and cost effectiveness of care, they could also be used for rationing" (Haines 1992: 785). Eddy who worked on new methods to develop guidelines confirmed that such fears are not too far-fetched. As he put it, outsiders might write "unnatural" policies that interfere with the "instincts" of physicians, taking over the control that used to lie within the medical profession: "While the use of policies as a management tool might have a desirable impact on quality of care and health care costs, it has several undesirable effects for practitioners. One is that it puts a mechanism designed for internal use in the hands of 'outsiders', such as utilization reviewers, the government, and insurers. Not only does this expose internal thoughts to external scrutiny, it opens those thoughts to manipulation. There is a concern that outsiders might write unnatural policies that do not match the instincts of practitioners. (...). But the greatest concern pertains to control. It is not stretching things too far to say that whoever controls practice policies controls medicine. That control used to lie exclusively, if diffusely, within the medical profession" (1990b: 880).

Given the divergent aims and rationalities of the different actors supporting guidelines, it becomes less surprising that practicing physicians, according to their own divergent aims and rationalities, may hesitate or resist applying it. When a physician in a treatment-decision with a patient neglects the suggestions given in a guideline, his/her reason may range from sheer ignorance over concrete reasons related to the specific case to conscious or unconscious resistance against the formalization and external control of medical practice. Considering the various motives that lie behind the introduction of guidelines, not only the practicing physician has "non-scientific" motives when not following treatment guidelines. Rather, guidelines and other instruments of Evidence-Based Medicine themselves also reflect the "non-scientific" motives of the different actors who demand and support their use in medical practice.

In the case of HIV/AIDS in Switzerland, guidelines are written and used mainly with the aim to increase the quality of treatment whereas cost-effectiveness or legal aspects are not central topics. Accordingly, physicians in our interviews discussed Evidence-Based Medicine and guidelines mainly as a specific source and type of knowledge which may question their personal knowledge. As the demand to treat patients in accordance with the guidelines gained legitimacy through the new treatment possibilities, some physicians feared their freedom of decision to be limited to the scope given in the guidelines, their work to be narrowed to the mere implementation of scientific research in practice, and their role to be reduced to an interface between medical science and the patient. Paradoxically, the very new treatment possibilities that relieved some physicians from their inability to act when con-

fronted with HIV patients thus meant for others a potential limitation in their freedom of decision-making. Medical uncertainty, often perceived as a burden for
individual decision-making, may in this context receive a liberating potential, as
described in chapter 6.6., by symbolizing the limits of scientific evidence and thus
supporting freedom of decision-making.

A remarkable form reflecting the ambivalent position and use of Evidence-Based
Medicine comes from a professor of clinical pharmacology who cast his arguments
in a dialogue between "Socrates" and "Enthusiasticus" (the latter representing Evidence-Based Medicine). In the course of the dialogue, Socrates shows sympathy for
the aims of Enthusiasticus, but he points out that Enthusiasticus moves away from
the reality of the practicing physician – and thus from the diversity of medical practice, which, as he implies, might not be formalized – since as a researcher he lacks
the time to practice medicine himself:

> "Socrates: (...) You must see that if you yourself are not constantly versed in the infi-
> nite variables of patient presentation and response to treatment, and dealing with them
> every day, you will be prey to criticism from those who do[158].
>
> Enthusiasticus: I have recently become aware of that and I am unsure how to deal with
> it. The matter is particularly acute because the cause of evidence based medicine has
> been taken up by those who manage our medical practice.
>
> Socrates: What is their interest?
>
> Enthusiasticus: They are particularly anxious to get value for money and wish to be
> sure that doctors' actions are effective and worth paying for.
>
> (...)
>
> Socrates: (...) {A}re you sure that the motives of the managers are as pure and intel-
> lectual as you imagine?
>
> Enthusiasticus: How could it be otherwise?
>
> Socrates: Is it not a manager's job to ensure that health care is delivered in the most
> cost-effective way possible? And do not all politicians exhort purchasers to get the best
> bargain?
>
> Enthusiasticus: Indeed.
>
> Socrates: Then what do you perceive as the main barrier to their purpose?
>
> Enthusiasticus: Lack of evidence as to what is really effective.
>
> Socrates: It would be nice, Enthusiasticus, my gullible friend, if it were really so, but I
> doubt it. The main barrier they perceive is an anarchic medical profession spending
> their money in a profligate and unnecessary manner. They see your beloved evidence
> based medicine as a means to shackle the doctors and bend them to their will. That, I
> am certain, is why they are so enthusiastic about it. Beware, Enthusiasticus, that you

---

[158] An argument which brings us back to the self-presentation of the founders of Evidence-Based Medicine, who, as outlined in chapter 6.2., keep emphasizing their own identity and career as medical practitioners.

are not used as a dupe in a political game of health economics. Remember, hemlock
may be down the line." (Grahame-Smith 1995: 1127)[159]

The author presents "Enthusiasticus" as a rather naïve but well-meaning character whose purpose is taken over and abused by managers and politicians who want
to control the anarchic physician according to their will. He thus provides a
dichotomous description of the noble intentions of the representative of Evidence-
Based Medicine whose purpose is taken over by managers and politicians who want
"to shackle the doctors and bend them to their will". Such an unfriendly takeover of
Evidence-Based Medicine may indeed reflect part of its history. Yet to some degree
it is contradicted by the view of external control and rationalization as inherent to
any formal codification of specialized knowledge (Turner 1995). Gordon (1988) for
example pointed out that the use of scientific data which claim universal validity
inevitably makes the physician's performance subject to external evaluation and
control. As the patient became visible to medicine, the physician and his/her practice
currently become visible and subject to economic and legal control.

Turner constructed a causal chain between systematic knowledge, the formal
codification of this knowledge, the establishment of routine practices, and the development of mechanisms for external control: "The basis of professional knowledge is
cognitive rationality whereby the privileged status of the profession is grounded in a
scientific discipline. However, this special and systematic body of knowledge also
provides the basis for external intervention and social control of the profession
itself. Where this knowledge can be codified and developed by computer systems[160],

---

[159] Copyright © 1995; *British Medical Journal*; reproduced here by kind permission of *British Medical
Journal*.

[160] Biomedical knowledge indeed has already become codified in computer programs that are intended
to take over part of the work of the practicing physician. For example, the HIV Medication Guide
(found on the Internet under http://www.jag.on.ca/hiv) "now includes over 350 drugs involved in the
management of HIV and opportunistic infections. Health care professionals as well as patients can
quickly design a medication administration schedule that reflects and can be integrated in someone's
routine. Each schedule is automatically checked for drug interactions against a very up-to-date bank of
over 650 interactions" (Therrien et al. 1998). The pharmaceutical companies *Glaxo Wellcome* and *Bio-
Chem Pharma* support the program.
Although such programs may still be of marginal use in practice, the authors proudly declared:
"program users from HIV clinics had been identified in Canada, the United States, Brazil, and Germany". Potential resistance against the program by physicians who may fear to be replaced by a computer was countered by the reassurance that the "HIV Medication Guide" cannot replace the physician.
According to Forsythe (1992) who did ethnographic research in artificial intelligence laboratories developing medical computer systems, part of the reason that computer systems are not well accepted by
medical practitioners lies in how user acceptance is evaluated. As researchers designing user evaluation
of these programs are committed to the values of the natural sciences, they try to choose methods of
evaluation that explicitly exclude users' subjective perception of their systems. They thus fail to evaluate
exactly the subjective resistance of potential users against their programs and to take account of it in the
program design. Instead, blame for lack of user acceptance is shifted to the users, a mechanism
expressed for example in terms like "end-user failure".

the profession becomes vulnerable to the rationalization of knowledge. Where the knowledge of the profession is grounded in natural science, this knowledge can become the basis of routine practices. The consequence of this form of knowledge is the possible fragmentation of the profession and its external control by bureaucratic means. It is for this reason that Jamous and Peloille[161] argue that professions need a barrier to protect themselves from such routinization and this barrier is constituted by the indetermination of knowledge; the knowledge of the profession has to have a distinctive mystique which suggests that there is a certain professional attitude and competence which cannot be reduced merely to systematic and routinized knowledge" (Turner 1995: 133).

What Turner described as the counter-discourse of medical professionals against routinization and external control is embodied in the discourse around the "art" of medicine. Stressing the art of medicine is an attempt to demarcate areas of medicine which are beyond formalization and where external evaluation of decisions and performance is neither appropriate nor legitimate. As the place and legitimization of "science" and "art" are negotiated, they are further formalized and delimited from each other by their adherents in the attempt to extend or defend their respective terrain in medical practice. The claim to integrate science into medical practice and the defense of the art of medicine in reaction to it might thus ultimately strengthen the opposition between the two concepts. It therefore remains open if Evidence-Based Medicine's efforts to better integrate the two types of knowledge rather contribute to their distinction and polarization.

---

[161] Jamous and Peloille (1970)

# CHAPTER 7

# CONCLUSIONS

> "It is not news that medicine and all
> other health care areas are rapidly
> changing. ('The future is already here;
> it just isn't evenly distributed yet.')."
> (Sackett et al. 1997: 16)

While this book focuses on HIV/AIDS and its medical care, it reflects current shifts in the concepts of sickness and the body and in the organization of medicine. Given the rapid changes in the field of HIV/AIDS through the introduction of combination therapies, these shifts became articulated and negotiated through HIV and AIDS due to the fact that they were taking place at an increased speed and on a large scale. I thus aimed at giving an insight into these shifts from the particular point of view that the field of HIV/AIDS provided during what Koenig (1988) described as the experimental phase of treatment. Some of the themes I discussed in my study include the expansion of chronic sickness, the ambivalent embodiment of an asymptomatic condition for people confronted with it, patients' and physicians' struggles with autonomy and dependence in medicine, the role of the general practitioner in an increasingly specialized medicine, and the new importance of basic and clinical science in the work of the individual physician. In concluding my text, I reflect on the processes of linking ethnographic work to its broader, even global context before I take up some of the themes discussed in the previous chapters by focusing on changing power relations in the fields of HIV/AIDS and medicine.

As the study is based on ethnography, it is not a macro-level overview over HIV/AIDS or medicine. Instead, I followed the themes and discourses that crossed the research into various directions. While I started to look at how people with HIV and their physicians were trying to make sense of HIV and AIDS as it was continually redefined, I gradually traced some of the origins, the wider context and the consequences of their insights and ideas. I looked at how people with HIV reconstructed their identity in the face of the virus as an invisible agent within the body, and how their constructions of HIV and the body stand in a mutual relationship with the ones developed by biomedicine and its practitioners. "Biomedicine" in turn once more proved to be an inaccurate description since it cannot adequately be described in monolithic terms (DelVecchio Good 1995a). Instead, I showed its heterogeneity by following the transformations of biomedical knowledge and the tensions and struggles between the different actors involved. On a global level of scientific research, I described how HIV/AIDS was negotiated between different specialties, i.e. between virology and immunology. I followed "the traffic between research medicine and clinical practice" (DelVecchio Good 1995b: 469) as it occurred – with considerable involvement of and support by pharmaceutical companies – from global scientific research to the national centers of HIV, i.e. to specialized clinics and their physicians who in turn participate in commissions that for example set the national guidelines on HIV/AIDS treatment, and from these onward to general practitioners. In this traffic, the HIV clinics hold an ambiguous status; they engage both in research medicine and in clinical practice. They are on an international level the recipients of scientific knowledge (yet also participating in the production of part of this knowledge through their own research), while on a national level they are standard-makers of medical practice.

In doing ethnographic work on medical knowledge, I focused on the processes that Hess (1992) emphasized as a specific and new contribution of anthropologists to studies of science and technology. These studies initially focused on the production of scientific facts in the laboratory, most prominently with the study by Latour and Woolgar (1986) first appearing in 1979. Starting around the late 1980s and early 1990s, anthropologists' ethnographies were "decentering the laboratory and transforming it into just one of the 'scenes' or 'sites' for the ethnography of science and technology" (Hess 1992: 14). In doing so, they were shifting the attention "from the *social construction* of scientific facts in laboratories (or artifacts in production settings) to the *cultural reconstruction* of scientific discourses and technical artifacts as they diffuse through scientific and nonscientific communities" (ibid.: 15, emphases in original). With this new focus, anthropologists were for example following medical knowledge as it diffused from laboratories and industry to the affected segments of the general public, or in the opposite direction, as exemplified by Martin (1994), they followed the roads by which cultural understandings transform knowledge within the laboratory.

"Following the roads" of themes and discourses may not only be understood metaphorically, but also literally, as again exemplified best by Martin's research on the immune system. When Marcus traced the emergence of "multi-sited ethnography", he praised Martin's research as "in a sense, the most fully achieved and rationalized multi-sited ethnography" (1995: 108). He further located examples of multi-sited ethnography mainly in a number of interdisciplinary fields of research that have evolved over the past decades, including specifically science and technology studies. In his definition, multi-sited research "is designed around chains, paths, threads, conjunctions, juxtapositions of locations in which the ethnographer establishes some form of literal, physical presence, with an explicit, posited logic of associations or connections among sites that in fact defines the argument of the ethnography" (ibid.: 105). In following the ideas about the immune system, Martin located her research in settings as diverse as, amongst others, an allergy clinic, a support group for survivors of polio, training courses for workers and managers, and alternative health clinics. As she vividly proved with her research, there are "a range of consequences that can be associated with transgressing the boundaries or stretching the limits of the 'field'" (Martin 1997: 134), since it was only by such transgression and stretching that she felt able to trace the "discontinuous, nonlinear, fractured ways that might link the citadel {of science} to the rest of the world" (ibid.: 136).

As I followed the roads of my study, I did not do so through a multi-sited approach. Rather, I was mainly located in a single site, although the research involved interviews (which required our presence) and questionnaires (filled out without our physical presence) with people located in diverse settings, and I did some mini-ethnographic work in other sites such as in conferences. To some degree, my ethnography might be framed by what Marcus called the "strategically situated single-site ethnography", which he characterized by the way the local situation is linked to other sites through the awareness and actions of people studied: "The key question is perhaps: What among locally probed subjects is iconic with or parallel to the identifiable similar or same phenomenon within the idioms and terms of another related or 'worlds apart' site? Answering this question involves the work of comparative translation and tracing among sites, which I suggested were basic to the methodology of multi-sited ethnography. Within a single site, the crucial issue concerns the detectable system-awareness in the everyday consciousness and actions of subjects' lives. This is not an abstract theoretical awareness such as a social scientist might seek, but a sensed, partially articulated awareness of specific other sites and agents to which particular subjects have (not always tangible) relationships" (ibid.: 110-111)[162].

Detecting and following what is "iconic with" or "parallel to" processes happening both within the realms of my research and in worlds apart, developing on the "system-awareness" of our interview partners, is how I composed my text. My approach thus can be envisioned as a radial one: If the empirical research is seen as the center, then different themes emerging from it are followed and are articulated to

---

[162] In emphasizing the "system-awareness in the everyday consciousness and actions of subjects' lives", Marcus evokes the theories developed by Bourdieu (1976) and by Giddens (1984) to overcome the dichotomy between actor and structure.

broader discourses. They thus spread out like roads from the center into various directions, but they always remain connected to it. Obviously, if such an approach is chosen, then it cannot be pre-determined exactly what the themes and discourses, or the roads followed, will be that finally come together in the text. While I started with an idea as narrow as investigating explanatory models of HIV among people living with it and health care providers, I ended in themes as diverse as for example scientific controversies, representations of antiretroviral medication by pharmaceutical companies, the role of the general practitioner in an increasingly specialized medicine, or the role of the state in controlling medicine.

The main advantages of such an open process of developing from the initial research to the final text are quite obvious. Firstly, it allows for the unexpected. In fact, to a certain degree the unexpected becomes the guiding principle in writing up the text. Secondly, it allows taking the complexity and global integration of the modern world into account. While some people with HIV may get their information on treatment from the Internet and their physicians may travel around the world to conferences or perform meta-analyses that integrate the findings of clinical trials performed in numerous sites across the world (yet, importantly, many other people with HIV and physicians for various reasons are *not* doing so), the ethnographer refraining from exploring such roads becomes an anachronism.

Yet there are also some problems to be considered when choosing such an approach. First of all, which themes do I write up from the abundance of material produced in any ethnography? It is tempting to borrow a concept prominent in medicine and to speak of the "art" of anthropology and the "intuition" of the anthropologist guiding this process, thus of an inexplicable and individual process. There is, of course, as much truth as rhetoric to this explanation as there is to the "art" of medicine. It is less mystifying to simply speak of the personal interest in and fascination with specific themes as a selection principle. Yet another selection principle not to be underestimated is what is defined as fashionable – and thus is written about – in the academic discourse. As it is the case in medicine, there are also global cultural centers of standard-making in anthropology, and in either case they are localized mainly in the global political and economic hegemonic centers. As much as "{d}ominant biotechnical societies, such as the United States, export not only medical knowledge, through direct training, scientific discourse (publications, meetings, international clinical trials), and medical products, but also a culture of biomedical practice" (DelVecchio Good 1995a: 200), these very societies also export through anthropological knowledge, discourses, and publications the dominant culture of anthropology. This fact explains why a research project which is, like mine, mainly conducted in Switzerland does not only refer to medical discourses mainly conducted in and emanating from the United States, but also to anthropological discourses from the same country[163].

A second problem related to a research approach as I chose it lies in delimiting the process of writing up. How broadly and how far away from my initial fieldwork and research questions do I trace the themes I write up? Setting the limits is not only an inevitably arbitrary act, a feature probably shared with all types of anthropological writing, but given the variety of the roads followed off the research site, many of them remain only superficially explored. Ideally, and this is the point where my research might fruitfully be carried further, some of these roads would lead to the discovery of new research sites and thus to a truly multi-sited ethnography. In the case of my study, such sites where the new era of AIDS is negotiated might for example include the public relations department of a pharmaceutical company, an AIDS hospice struggling with the decreasing number of patients, or the public health department of a resource-poor country fighting to gain access to antiretroviral medication.

Yet, as the above-mentioned example of the Internet paradigmatically shows, the very definition of an ethnographic "site", or a "field", is increasingly problematic. Not only are their boundaries permeable, but also they are not necessarily linked to physical localities anymore. Where, for example, is the Internet? Where do I go to investigate the sources of information people get from it? Of course, I might do

---

[163] In fact, as an anthropologist living if certainly not in the global economic periphery, then certainly in the anthropological periphery, I am struck when reading how few leading anthropologists from the center care to challenge the global hegemonic structure of our discipline. In "The Predicament of Culture", James Clifford (1988) claimed to have challenged ethnographic authority, yet explicitly limited his discussion to English, American and French ethnographic writing while assuming that his observations could be generalized to other disciplinary traditions. George Marcus found it to be "perhaps no accident that exemplars thus far of multi-sited fieldwork have been developed in monolingual (largely Anglo-American) contexts in which fine-grained knowledge of the language is unproblematic for native English speakers. Yet, if such ethnography is to flourish in arenas that anthropology has defined as emblematic interests, it will soon have to become as multilingual as it is multi-sited" (1995: 101). He neither developed ideas on how multi-sited ethnography should become multilingual, nor did he explain why he assumed the anthropologist to be a native English speaker. Gupta and Ferguson limited their reader, similar to Clifford, mainly to "mainstream social/cultural anthropology as practiced in leading departments in the United States and the United Kingdom" (1997: 1). Unlike Clifford a decade earlier, they did not claim that this focus could be generalized, and they seemed to feel a need for justification. They justified their focus with the very hegemonic structures in anthropology – whose mechanisms they aptly summarize – which led them to choose it: "Our focus on what one might call the hegemonic centers of the discipline is deliberate and motivated. Since we are concerned, above all, with the mechanisms through which dominant disciplinary norms and conventions are established, we believe there is good reason for paying special attention to those institutional sites and national contexts that, in practice, enjoy a disproportionate say in setting theoretical and methodological agendas and defining what will (and will not) count as 'real anthropology,' not only in the U.S. or U.K., but throughout the anthropological world" (ibid.: 40).

fieldwork at a particular provider's, or in a group running a specific homepage concerning my research topic, but does this capture what people mean when they speak of the relevance of "the Internet" for their work or lives? Isn't it even besides the point to locate specific sites for research when the Internet is characterized exactly by being nowhere physically and yet, given the infrastructure, potentially accessible from everywhere? Clifford wondered if an "electronic travel" into the Internet would count as fieldwork: "What if someone studied the culture of computer hackers (a perfectly acceptable anthropology project in many, if not all, departments) and in the process never 'interfaced' in the flesh with a single hacker. Would the months, even years, spent on the Net be fieldwork?" (1997: 192). Asking his colleagues, he found that most of them would count it as fieldwork, but they would hesitate to supervise a Ph.D. dissertation based primarily on such fieldwork which is still too unorthodox to pass as anthropological research.

In a similarly vein to the Internet, other fields also seem to denote imaginary locations rather than geographical, physical localities. Where is a specific scientific discipline located? Or, does "the field of HIV/AIDS" refer to specific localities? I may trace them in conferences, labs, universities, and study the texts, objects, images used and produced there. But do I thus capture the rapid, transnational circulation of thoughts and things, which in most cases does not even require physical mobility, that increasingly characterizes any scientific discipline or any phenomenon as complex as HIV/AIDS? While Marcus stated that multi-sited ethnography arose mainly "in response to empirical changes in the world and therefore to transformed locations of cultural production" (1995: 97), one wonders if these very empirical changes and transformed locations that require multi-sited approaches might at the same time make them partly obsolete or impossible by diminishing the importance of the physical locality both of the subject under study and the ethnographer as determining their participation in a specific site, and by increasingly creating sites not physically located. Whereas the anthropological "field", denoting the site where anthropological fieldwork takes place, still has the implicit connotations of a clearance in an agrarian, set apart, even wild (Gupta and Ferguson 1997) or, at least, muddy (Clifford 1997) place, entire fields and their cultural dynamics increasingly become deterriorialized (Appadurai 1991). Gupta and Ferguson suggested that anthropologist should try to redefine their sites and fields, a redefinition that they described as a shift from "locality" to "location": "Ethnography's great strength has always been its explicit and well-developed sense of location, of being set-here-and-not-elsewhere. This strength becomes a liability when notions of 'here' and 'elsewhere' are assumed to be features of geography, rather than sites constructed in fields of unequal power relations" (1997: 35). They thus see the anthropologist's location firstly as a site not given but constructed, and secondly as located within fields which seem to come close to the notion of the field developed by Bourdieu rather than to the muddy clearance envisioned in anthropological fieldwork. In

Bourdieu's concept, the field is a sub-division of the social world which is defined not by spatial locality, but by having its own institutions, rules, values, and objects of interests which are to some degree shared, but also fought over by its actors, and whose structure reflects the power relations between these actors (Bourdieu 1993).

The power relations in the field of HIV/AIDS, or more precisely the changes in power relations brought about by or accentuated through the introduction of new treatment options, are indeed a main underlying theme that links the different roads I followed in order to describe the new era of AIDS. As I take up in the following paragraphs of my conclusions a few of the themes discussed in the previous chapters, I therefore focus on showing how the changes in the field of HIV/AIDS partly cause, partly highlight changes in power relations between the actors involved and reflect broader changes in power relations in medicine. In focusing on changing power relations, I largely depart, as many others do, from a notion of power as Foucault has elaborated it. In the following, I mostly draw upon his emphasis on power as multi-sited, heterogeneous, and diverse, since it reflects the situation I found in my research. Power in Foucault's perspective is not a superstructure; instead, relations of power are everywhere (Gordon 1980). Power is manifold; there is not one power, but various combinations and hierarchies of powers that work on different levels. They may be combined, they may inhibit and neutralize each other, they may reinforce each other. Different forms and combinations of powers thus have to be analyzed in their unique manifestations (Foucault 1999). I believe that ethnography with its tradition of developing its analysis from fieldwork (whatever the field may be), and thus ideally from detailed and intimate knowledge of specific social situations, provides a promising background to accomplish this task. Such an ethnographic approach though has to omit what Bourdieu and Wacquant (2000) called the tendency in the social sciences to replace the analysis of structures and mechanisms of power through a mystification of the culture and the point of view of the people who are excluded from that power. I hope that by continuously linking the local situations I encountered to global processes – and vice versa – I have not fallen into this trap.

Common to our interview partners – persons with HIV as well as their physicians – is the remarkable easiness in combining different concepts in explaining the onset, course, and consequences of HIV. The infection is as much framed in terms of a virus and the immune system interacting with each other (a framework which, as I have tried to outline, is far from being as value-free and uncontested as its constructors would have it), as it is a social sickness, an expression of a disruption of the social relations of the individual infected as well as a disruption within society as a whole. In making sense of HIV, people have to face and integrate different perspectives, from existential questions to day-to-day decisions, and it seems only sensible to refer to different kinds of rationality, to employ different versions of reasoning (Hunt and Mattingly 1998). While science still struggles with overcoming basic Western assumptions such as mind/body and self/other dichotomies (Lock 1993a), our interview partners easily transgressed these boundaries by describing the interrelation between mind and body in the course of their sickness or by attributing sickness as much to the interaction between the virus and the immune system as to malevolent social relations. They thus combined externalizing explanations concentrating on the etiology of sickness, commonly attributed to cultures and societies lacking our individualized conception of the body-self, with the internalizing explanations closer to biomedicine and more desired in Western societies (Helman 1994; Scheper-Hughes and Lock 1987).

People with HIV are certainly the ones whose lives became most dramatically changed through the introduction of the new antiretroviral medications. As also scientists and physicians did, people confronted with a positive HIV test had come to view the infection as an ultimately deadly condition with limited treatment opportunities. Under the condition of therapeutic impotence, they struggled to assume responsibility for and control over their condition. Given the lack of efficient treatment, they inevitably relied on strategies of self-control, most notably through changes in attitude and lifestyle. Such strategies largely follow, though from the point of view of people who had crossed the line between the healthy and the infected, a middle-class attitude of health as a good to be achieved through self-control (Crawford 1985; 1994).

With the new treatment opportunities, these strategies increasingly became questioned. The introduction of combination therapies profoundly changed health care in HIV, both when patients take therapies as well as when they are not taking them. While living without medical treatment was formerly more or less a taken for granted situation for asymptomatic people, it now turned into a decision to be taken, a decision that might itself become a new stigma. The mere possibility of treatment, and even more so the decision to take treatment, imply that own measures to control the infection have become obsolete and are replaced by a medical product. Treatment thus may threaten the integrity and autonomy achieved in a long personal process. On a physical level, the medication receives a status similar to the virus itself, entering the body as an unknown factor from the outside and acting unpredictably within the body. Medication thus turns into a new and powerful actor, a status actively promoted by pharmaceutical companies, and its power may be hoped for and yet feared. On the social level, treatment means increased dependence on the health care system, including its practitioners and the technical devices that produce, for example, the laboratory data which largely guide treatment. While the power to control the infection shifts to the medication and the health care system, patients' responsibility nevertheless turns into a central element of health care professionals' discourse. Given the uncertainty of treatment and the difficulties of its regimen, this discourse centers on the role of patients in the treatment-decision and in treatment adherence. As the legitimacy to control the HIV infection thus becomes the domain of medicine, the responsibility for the treatment decision and outcome to some degree remains the domain of the patient.

Physicians took different positions vis-à-vis the new treatment according to their own position within the field of medicine. Uncertainty concerning the onset, course, and efficacy of treatment, in a situation when guidelines were constantly changing and no long-term experience was yet available, allowed for an open negotiation of treatment decisions between doctor and patient. The fluctuating situation thus reinforced what many physicians see as their role and strength in the health care system, namely advocating the patient's view and supporting patients' own decision-making on care and cure. The role of the patient as an equal partner in health care decisions though remains partial and is an ambiguous one. Firstly, physicians tend to limit patient autonomy in those fields where they see their own strengths and competencies. HIV specialists who are closer to the sources of new knowledge on treatment may be more inclined to shape the patient's treatment decision. Meanwhile, with the increasing complexity of treatment, general practitioners move further away from the curing aspects of health care. In compensation, they tend to emphasize what they and their patients often see as the generalists' strength in health care, i.e. providing continuity of care and an ongoing doctor-patient relationship. Given this emphasis, they may for example disapprove of patients' autonomy in freely combining different health care providers through health care shopping. Secondly, stressing the patient's active, responsible role in health care may be, as outlined above, a strategy to compensate for the uncertainties in HIV treatment. Liberating the patient from a paternalistic interaction thus also means sharing the uncertainty of and the responsibility for the long-term outcome of treatment. Thirdly, as emphasized by practically all physicians and belonging to the standard medical discourse on antiretroviral treatment, basing treatment on patients' decisions is inevitable to carry through a complex and demanding long-term treatment. In that sense, patient choice may be in some instances an inevitable rather than a desired aspect of the doctor-patient interaction. Fourthly, stressing a symmetrical relationship in the doctor-patient interaction may compensate for new asymmetrical power relations the practicing physician is faced with in medicine. Various actors, including specialized physicians, medical associations, insurance companies or government representatives make new claims to monitor and influence medical practice. In this situation, physicians – especially but not exclusively general practitioners – may increasingly face their loss of power and authority and find themselves in a structurally inferior position similar to the one of the patient. Stressing patients' preferences may become a strategy to defend individual decision-making and variety in clinical practice against intra- and extra-professional claims to control or standardize medical practice.

Given the ambiguous aims and motives for a more egalitarian, less paternalistic doctor-patient interaction and the increasing importance of actors standing behind the practicing physician, patient empowerment within the doctor-patient interaction runs the risk of leaving the main arenas of medical decision-making unchallenged. The doctor-patient interaction to a decreasing degree reflects the locus where power is enacted and negotiated in medicine. Instead, I argue that the most pronounced changes in medical power are found in the relations between specialists and generalists as well as in the interaction between clinical science and clinical practice. Both of these fields are in turn partly linked to a changing relationship of the medical profession with its political and economic partners.

In the case of HIV, the autonomy of the practicing physician is negotiated mainly through the role attributed to specialist consultations and treatment guidelines in treatment decisions. They received new importance and provoked new controversies with the introduction of combination therapies. On an institutional level, the specialized HIV centers became more influential as their physicians possess the knowledge – provisional as it always is – on the complicated treatment regimens. The controversial relationship between general practitioners and HIV specialists was represented through the discussions led in medical journals around revised care schemes in the era of combination therapies and through physicians' emotional statements on the collaboration across the generalist-specialist boundary. As stories about losing patients to the HIV centers when sharing care illustrate, the role allocation between generalists and specialists also entails concrete economic implications along with the struggle over knowledge, competence, and ultimately power, which in turn characterizes medicine as a whole.

Knowledge and competence do not simply leave the domain of the general practitioner to be placed in the hands of the specialist. They also, as illustrated by the new status of guidelines, more radically slip out of the control of the practicing physician. The key term around which this trend crystallizes is "Evidence-Based Medicine", a movement that aims at further integrating external evidence into the physician's work. With meta-analyses, systematic reviews and evidence-based guidelines, Evidence-Based Medicine provides the methods and tools for a new step in the rationalization of medical knowledge. While the experience of the individual physician in patient care is explicitly acknowledged as a basis for implementing the data provided by Evidence-Based Medicine, the exponents of Evidence-Based Medicine just as explicitly question and challenge the common idea that individual expertise and competence increase with experience. In fact, if expertise and competence are defined as the "knowledge of up-to-date care" (Sackett et al. 1997: 9) according to the standards of Evidence-Based Medicine, then increasing experience leads to decreasing expertise and competence in clinical practice. Basic to such an argument is a redefinition and, most importantly, a relocation of medical knowledge. With the increasingly sophisticated methods of data gathering (i.e. the double-blind controlled clinical trial) and processing (i.e. meta-analyses and systematic reviews), medical science gains further terrain and legitimacy as the source of medical knowledge. In the old debate about the respective roles of science and art in medicine, the scope of art as the personal knowledge of the physician thus becomes further limited. What is defined as legitimate knowledge is increasingly dissociated from the person of the physician and allocated instead somewhere "out there" in the world of science where acquiring it is primarily a matter of methods.

With the decreasing legitimacy of the individual physician's expertise, his/her role is increasingly narrowed to an interface between science and the patient. Thus, while much research focuses on the asymmetry and dependence between patient and physician, there is indeed a formal analogy in their situation. Physicians, especially general practitioners which "are often considered the end users of evidence-based medicine after it has trickled down from researchers and hospital specialists" (Smith et al. 2000: 42), seem to be just as anxious about re-establishing boundaries and keeping independence and control as their patients are. Their boundaries to be defended run between individual expertise and scientific evidence, between autonomy and external control, and in the case of general practitioners, between general and specialized medicine. Not surprisingly though, also physicians – again in analogy to their patients – develop counter-discourses and -strategies against the standardization, rationalization, and control of health care. In many instances, they are supported by the physicians favoring and representing Evidence-Based Medicine and guidelines yet rejecting their use as means of external economic and legal control of medicine. On the one hand, physicians explicitly fraternize with their patients by arguing with patient preferences and the necessary adaptation of guidelines to their patients' individual situations as a central element of health care. On the other hand, they question scientific evidence by arguing with its very limits, i.e. with the uncertainty paradoxically resulting from the continuing expansion of knowledge and from the deficiencies of this knowledge, which may not meet the methodological standards set by Evidence-Based Medicine. Linking the scientific power of knowledge to its legitimacy in controlling medical practice is also reflected for example in the argumentation of Woolf, an adherent of guidelines, who proposed "a model that would link the intensity of enforcement to the scientific and clinical quality of the practice guidelines" (1993: 2652).

Defining who produces, holds, and disseminates the relevant knowledge in medicine is similar to the allocation of roles between patients and physicians and between generalists and specialists, intrinsically interwoven with struggles around the association between power and knowledge. Following Foucault, these struggles reflect the opposition against the types of power which are linked to knowledge, competence, and formal qualifications, and which Foucault called the "regime of knowledge" (1999: 166). The struggles are carried out between patients and physicians in the medical encounter, between physicians of different specialties and of different positions in relation to medical science as well as between physicians or physician associations and economic and political actors in the field of medicine. The emotional and controversial discussions of patient autonomy vs. physician authority, of science and art in medicine, of guidelines, of Evidence-Based Medicine, as well as of care schemes that try to allocate generalists' and specialists' roles and responsibilities in patient care must be placed within this framework. They do not represent value-free concepts and instruments, and neither are they perceived as such by the actors confronted with them.

Unraveling the various and often divergent rationalities, aims, and interests of the different actors that crossed my research was, as I have come to believe retrospectively, indeed the main motive to write this book. Walking back and forth between anthropology and medicine, I hope to have taken advantage of what I described in the introduction as a liminal position in order to do so. Following the inspiring variety of ideas and the motives of different actors and showing how they are negotiated, often departing from uneven power relations, appears to me as a fruitful way to trace the processes of change captured in this research. But why would such an ethnography of change matter? Turner believed that "the development of the AIDS epidemic is clearly a major transformation of the character and significance of disease in contemporary society" (1995: 218). I might add that the AIDS epidemic not only transformed and keeps transforming the character and significance of disease (and its interaction with the body), but also of medicine and health care. An ethnographic approach to these processes inevitably shows that they are not only complex, but sometimes even paradoxical: As people with HIV fear losing responsibility for and control over their infection through antiretroviral therapies' "promise of power"[164] promoted by pharmaceutical companies, medical practitioners facing uncertainty stress their patients' responsibilities in deciding for treatment and controlling it through adherence. While medicine gains back power through the introduction of treatment, physicians may through the very same process fear losing their autonomy by having to narrow their work to the implementation of guidelines. These guidelines, which stand for the new power of clinical science in medical practice, in turn also reflect the processes by which the medical profession is increasingly controlled by economic and political actors. While the new era of AIDS thus may easily be interpreted as a paradigm for the "insatiable appetite for medical products and services which has produced a global market for the medical profession whose social power has been correspondingly enhanced" (Turner 1995: 233), it just as easily exemplifies the diminishing power and autonomy of the medical profession struggling against extra-professional interference.

---

[164] As *Roche* advertised *Saquinavir* (*POZ Magazine*, Issue 37, July 1998, p. 114). See chapter 4.2.

I have shown that broad changes in the meaning of sickness and the body, in the roles of patients and practitioners in health care, and in the definition, production and diffusion of knowledge in medicine are both exemplified and co-constructed in the field of HIV/AIDS. These changes though, as the above paradoxes indicate, are multi-faceted and do not lead to a single direction. Living in a complex world, I do not assume that highlighting some of these facets will eventually provide a broad and coherent picture. Instead, it helps to expose some of the rhetoric used, to see some of the intended and unintended consequences, to understand some of the complex interrelations of seemingly independent developments, and to ask new questions.

# REFERENCES

Abbott, A. "The European pharmaceutical outlook." *Nature* 361.6414 (1993): 765-768.

Albert, E. "Illness and deviance: the response of the press to AIDS." In *The social dimension of AIDS*, edited by D. I. Feldman and T. M. Johnson, 163-178. New York: Praeger, 1986.

Altorfer, R. ""Es geht um die Glaubwürdigkeit als Hausärzte"." *Ars Medici* 10 (1997): 579-579.

Annas, G. J. "Reframing the debate on health care reform by replacing our metaphors." *New England Journal of Medicine* 332.11 (1995): 744-747.

Anonymous. "Empathy: can it be taught?" *Annals of Internal Medicine* 117.8 (1992): 700-701.

Anonymous. "Recruitment and funding: special feature." *Nature* 361.6414 (1993): 757.

Appadurai, A. "Global ethnoscapes. Notes and queries for a transnational anthropology." In *Recapturing anthropology*, edited by R. G. Fox, 191-210. Santa Fe: School of American Research Press, 1991.

Arbeitskreis HIV. "Angst ist der Killer." *Angst In Dir Selbst AIDS* (1996): 17.

Ariss, R. M., and G. W. Dowsett. *Against death. The practice of living with AIDS*. Amsterdam: Gordon and Breach, 1997.

Atkinson, P. *Medical talk and medical work. The liturgy of the clinic*. London: Sage Publications, 1995.

Baker, A. J. "The portrayal of AIDS in the media: an analysis of articles in the New York Times." In *The social dimension of AIDS*, edited by D. I. Feldman and T. M. Johnson, 179-193. New York: Praeger, 1986.

Baltimore, D. "Lessons from people with nonprogressive HIV infection." *New England Journal of Medicine* 332.4 (1995): 259-260.

Bassetti, S., M. Battegay, H. Furrer, et al. "Why is highly active antiretroviral therapy (HAART) not prescribed or discontinued?" *Journal of Acquired Immune Deficiency Syndromes and Human Retrovirology* 21.2 (1999): 114-119.

Bayer, R. "Public health policy and the AIDS epidemic: an end to HIV exceptionalism." *New England Journal of Medicine* 324.21 (1991): 1500-1504.

Bayer, R., and G. Oppenheimer. AIDS, death, and impotence: doctors confront the limits of medicine. AIDS in Europe, Paris (1998): Sy 9.1.

Beisecker, A. E., and T. D. Beisecker. "Using metaphors to characterize doctor-patient relationships: paternalism versus consumerism." *Health Communication* 5.1 (1993): 41-58.

Benoist, J. "Le médicament, opérateur technique et médiateur symbolique." *Médecine et anthropologie* 1 (1989/1990): 45-50.

Benoist, J., and P. Cathebras. "The body: from one immateriality to another." *Social Science and Medicine* 36.7 (1993): 857-865.

Benoist, J., and A. Desclaux. "Pour une anthropologie impliquée." In *Anthropologie et sida. Bilan et perspectives*, edited by J. Benoist and A. Desclaux, 363-373. Paris: Editions Karthala, 1996.

Bobbio, M., B. Demichelis, and G. Giustetto. "Completeness of reporting trial results: effect on physicians' willingness to prescribe." *The Lancet* 343.8907 (1994): 1209-1211.

Bodenheimer, T. S. "The transnational pharmaceutical industry and the health of the world's people." In *Issues in the political economy of health care*, edited by J. B. McKinlay, 187-216. New York: Tavistock, 1985.

Bommes, M., and A. Scherr. "Der Gebrauchswert von Selbst- und Fremdethnisierung in Strukturen sozialer Ungleichheit." *Prokla* 21.2 (1991): 291-316.

Boseley, S. "Struggle for cheap medicines. World Trade Organisation: special report." *The Guardian*, Nov. 27, 1999.

171

Bourdieu, P. *Entwurf einer Theorie der Praxis auf der Basis der ethnologischen Grundlage der kabylischen Gesellschaft.* Frankfurt a. M.: Suhrkamp, 1976.

Bourdieu, P. *Soziologische Fragen.* Frankfurt a. M.: Suhrkamp, 1993.

Bourdieu, P., and L. Wacquant. "Schöne neue Begriffswelt." *Le monde diplomatique,* Mai 2000, 7.

Bradley, C. B. "Uncomfortable prescribing decisions: a critical incident study." *British Medical Journal* 304.6822 (1992): 294-296.

Branch, W. T., R. A. Arky, B. Woo, et al. "Teaching medicine as a human experience: a patient-doctor relationship course for faculty and first-year medical students." *Annals of Internal Medicine* 114.6 (1991): 482-489.

Britten, N. "Patients' ideas about medicines: a qualitative study in a general practice population." *British Journal of General Practice* 44.387 (1994): 465-468.

Britten, N. "Patients' demands for prescriptions in primary care." *British Medical Journal* 310.6987 (1995a): 1084-1085.

Britten, N. "Qualitative interviews in medical research." *British Medical Journal* 311.6999 (1995b): 251-253.

Britten, N., and O. Okoumunne. "The influence of patients' hopes of receiving a prescription on doctors' perception and the decision to prescribe: a questionnaire survey." *British Medical Journal* 315.7121 (1997): 1506-1510.

Broers, B., A. Morabia, and B. Hirschel. "A cohort study of drug users' compliance with zidovudine treatment." *Archives of Internal Medicine* 154.10 (1994): 1121-1127.

Brunner, H. H. "GRAT-Projekt - Zielsetzungen und Geschichte." *Schweizerische Ärztezeitung* 78.21 (1997a): 775-777.

Brunner, H. H. "GRAT-Projekt - Zielsetzungen und Geschichte II." *Schweizerische Ärztezeitung* 78.24 (1997b): 895ff.

Bryman, A. *Quantity and quality in social research.* London: Unwin Hyman, 1988.

Buchbinder, S. P., M. H. Katz, N. A. Hessol, et al. "Long-term HIV-1 infection without immunological progression." *AIDS* 8.8 (1994): 1123-1128.

Bucher, H. C. "Evidence Based Medicine." *Ars Medici* 10 (1997): 591-596.

Bucher, H. C., M. Weinbacher, and K. Gyr. "Influence of method of reporting study results on decision of physicians to prescribe drugs to lower cholesterol concentration." *British Medical Journal* 309.6957 (1994): 761-764.

Bury, M. "Chronic illness as biographical disruption." *Sociology of Health and Illness* 4.2 (1982): 167-182.

Bury, M. "The sociology of chronic illness: a review of research and prospects." *Sociology of Health and Illness* 13.4 (1991): 451-468.

Byrne, S., and B. E. L. Long. *Doctors talking to patients.* London: Department of Health and Social Security, 1976.

Cao, Y., L. Qin, L. Zhang, et al. "Virologic and immunologic characterization of long-term survivors of Human Immunodeficiency Virus Type 1 infection." *New England Journal of Medicine* 332.4 (1995): 201-208.

Carricaburu, D., and J. Pierret. "From biographical disruption to biographical reinforcement: the case of HIV-positive men." *Sociology of Health and Illness* 17.1 (1995): 65-88.

Cassell, E. J. "Disease as "it": concepts of disease revealed by patients presenting symptoms." *Social Science and Medicine* 10.3-4 (1976a): 143-146.

Cassell, E. J. *The healer's art. A new approach to the doctor-patient relationship.* Philadelphia: Lippincott, 1976b.

Centers for Disease Control. "1993 revised classification system for HIV infection and expanded surveillance definition for AIDS among adolescents and adults." *MMWR Morbidity and Mortality Weekly Report* 41.ec 18 (1992): 1-19.

Chabot, J. M. "Spécial EBM." *Post-Scriptum - Lettre trimestrielle de l'analyse de la littérature internationale sur la formation et les pratiques médicales* 3 (1999): 1-4.

Chalmers, J., K. Dickersin, and T. C. Chalmers. "Getting to grips with Archie Cochrane's agenda." *British Medical Journal* 305.6857 (1992): 786-788.

Champaloux, B. "Les pratiques profanes de santé des personnes vivant avec le VIH." In *Anthropologie et sida. Bilan et perspectives*, edited by J. Benoist and A. Desclaux, 179-200. Paris: Editions Karthala, 1996.

Charbonney, R. "Adherence - Herausforderung für die Medizin." *Aids Infothek* 5 (1998): 4-12.

Chesney, M. A., and F. M. Hecht. Adherence to HIV antiretroviral therapy: an essential element to understanding treatment effect. AIDS in Europe, Paris (1998): Sy 5.2.

Chua-Eoan, H. "The tao of Ho." *Time*, December 30, 1996 / January 6, 1997, 39-40.

Clarke, A. "Barriers to general practitioners caring for patients with HIV/AIDS." *Family Practice* 10.1 (1993): 8-13.

Clarke, J. N. "Media portrayal of disease from the medical, political economy and lifestyle perspective." *Qualitative Health Research* 1.3 (1991): 287-308.

Clifford, J. *The predicament of culture. Twentieth-century ethnography, literature, and art.* Cambridge: Harvard University Press, 1988.

Clifford, J. "Spatial practices: fieldwork, travel, and the disciplining of anthropology." In *Anthropological locations: boundaries and grounds of a field science*, edited by A. Gupta and J. Ferguson, 185-222. Berkeley: University of California Press, 1997.

Cochrane, A. L. *Effectiveness and efficiency. Random reflections on health services.* London: Nuffield Provincial Hospitals Trust, 1972.

Cockburn, J., and S. Pit. "Prescribing behaviour in clinical practice: patients' expectations and doctors' perceptions of patients' expectations - a questionnaire study." *British Medical Journal* 315.7107 (1997): 520-523.

Cohen, J. "Exploring how to get at - and eradicate - hidden HIV." *Science* 279.5358 (1998): 1854-1855.

Condra, J. H., and E. A. Emini. "Preventing HIV-1 drug resistance." *Science & Medicine* 4.1 (1997).

Conrad, P. "The meaning of medication: another look at compliance." *Social Science and Medicine* 20.1 (1985): 29-37.

Conrad, P. "The experience of illness: recent and new directions." *Research in the Sociology of Health Care* 6 (1987): 1-31.

Conroy, M., and W. Shannon. "Clinical guidelines: their implementation in general practice." *British Journal of General Practice* 45.396 (1995): 371-375.

Corbin, J., and A. L. Strauss. "Accompaniments of chronic illness: changes in body, self, biography, and biographical time." *Research in the Sociology of Health Care* 6 (1987): 249-281.

Crawford, R. "A cultural account of "health": control, release, and the social body." In *Issues in the political economy of health care*, edited by J. B. McKinlay, 60-103. London: Tavistock, 1985.

Crawford, R. "The boundaries of the self and the unhealthy other: reflections on health, culture and AIDS." *Social Science and Medicine* 38.10 (1994): 1347-1365.

Dannecker, M. "Profanisierung von Aids durch die neuen Therapien." In *Neue Aids-Medikamente - neue ethische Probleme?*, edited by Aids Info Docu Schweiz, 12-18. Bern: Aids Info Docu Schweiz, 1997.

Davidoff, F., B. Haynes, D. Sackett, et al. "Evidence based medicine. A new journal to help doctors identify the information they need." *British Medical Journal* 310.6987 (1995): 1085-1086.

Davies, M. L. "Shattered assumptions: time and the experience of long-term HIV-positivity." *Social Science and Medicine* 44.5 (1997): 561-571.

Davis, D. A., M. A. Thompson, A. D. Oxman, et al. "Changing physician performance. A systematic review of the effect of continuing medical education strategies." *JAMA* 274.9 (1995): 700-705.

DelVecchio Good, M.-J. *American medicine: the quest for competence.* Berkeley: University of California Press, 1995a.

DelVecchio Good, M.-J. "Cultural studies of biomedicine: an agenda for research." *Social Science and Medicine* 41.4 (1995b): 461-473.

DelVecchio Good, M.-J., B. Good, C. Schaffer, et al. "American oncology and the discourse on hope." *Culture, Medicine, and Psychiatry* 14.1 (1990): 59-79.

Derber, C. "Physicians and their sponsors: the new medical relations of production." In *Issues in the political economy of health care*, edited by J. B. McKinlay, 217-254. New York: Tavistock, 1985.

Desclaux, A. Evaluation d'accompagnement de la multithérapie antiretrovirale chez les patients VIH 1 du Sénégal. Aspects sociaux et observance. Pré-enquête: PNLS Sénégal/IMEA/ORSTOM, Projet SIDAK AC 12, 1998.

DiGiacomo, S. M. "Metaphor as illness: postmodern dilemmas in the representation of body, mind and disorder." *Medical Anthropology* 14.1 (1992): 109-137.

DiGiacomo, S. M. "Can there be a "cultural epidemiology"?" *Medical Anthropology Quarterly* 13.4 (1999): 436-457.

Dong, K., M. M. Flynn, P. B. Dickinson, et al. Changes in body habitus in HIV (+) women after initiation with protease inhibitor therapy. 12th World AIDS Conference, Geneva (1998): 12373.

Donovan, J. L., and D. R. Blake. "Patient non-compliance: deviance or reasoned-decision-making?" *Social Science and Medicine* 34.5 (1992): 507-513.

Douglas, M. *Purity and danger: an analysis of the concepts of pollution and taboo.* London: Routledge and Kegan, 1966.

Duesberg, P. H. "Human Immunodeficiency Virus and Acquired Immunodeficiency Syndrome: correlation but not causation." *Proceedings of the National Academy of Sciences of the United States of America* 86.3 (1989): 755-764.

Durant, J. A new agenda for the public understanding of science, London, Imperial College (1995): Inaugural Lecture.

Dürst, M. "Stärken Sie Ihr Immunsystem." *Optima*, Mai 1999, 37-39.

Easterbrook, P. J. "Non-progression in HIV infection." *AIDS* 8.8 (1994): 1179-1182.

Eddy, D. M. "Designing a practice policy. Standards, guidelines, and options." *JAMA* 263.22 (1990a): 3077, 3081-3081.

Eddy, D. M. "Practice policies - what are they?" *JAMA* 263.6 (1990b): 877-878, 880.

Eddy, D. M. "Practice policies: where do they come from?" *JAMA* 263.9 (1990c): 1265, 1269, 1272, 1275.

Editorial. "Leap of faith over the data tap." *The Lancet* 345.8963 (1995): 1449-1451.

Editorial. "Sleep less in Seattle." *The Lancet* 354.9194 (1999): 1917.

Egger, M., B. Hirschel, P. Francioli, et al. "Impact of new antiretroviral combination therapies in HIV infected patients in Switzerland: prospective multicentre study." *British Medical Journal* 315.7117 (1997): 1194-1199.

Ellrodt, G., D. J. Cook, J. Lee, et al. "Evidence-based disease management." *JAMA* 278.20 (1997): 1687-1691.

Elmer-Dewitt, P. "Turning the tide." *Time*, December 30, 1996 / January 6, 1997, 26-51.

Erger, J., O. Grusky, T. Mann, et al. "HIV healthcare provider-patient interaction: observations on the process of providing antiretroviral treatment." *AIDS Patient Care and STDs* 14.5 (2000): 259-268.

Estroff, S. E. "Identity, disability, and schizophrenia: the problem of chronicity." In *Knowledge, power and practice: the anthropology of medicine and everyday life*, edited by S. Lindenbaum and M. Lock, 246-285. Berkeley: University of California Press, 1993.

Fauci, A. S. "Resistance to HIV-1 infection: it's in the genes." *Nature Medicine* 2.9 (1996): 966-967.

Fee, E., and N. Krieger. "Thinking and rethinking AIDS: implications for health policy." *International Journal of Health Services* 23.2 (1993a): 323-346.

Fee, E., and N. Krieger. "Understanding AIDS: historical interpretations and the limits of biomedical individualism." *American Journal of Public Health* 83.10 (1993b): 1477-1486.

Feinberg, M. B. "Guidelines for the use of antiretroviral agents in HIV-infected adults and adolescents." *MMWR Morbidity and Mortality Weekly Report* 47.RR-5 (1998): 43-65.

Feldman, J. "The French are different - French and American medicine in the context of AIDS." *Western Journal of Medicine* 157.3 (1992): 345-349.

Feldman, J. L. *Plague doctors: responding to the AIDS epidemic in France and America.* Westport: Bergin and Garvey, 1995.

Fisher, P., and A. Ward. "Complementary medicine in Europe." *British Medical Journal* 309.6947 (1994): 107-111.

Forrow, L., W. C. Taylor, and R. M. Arnold. "Absolutely relative: how research results are summarized can affect treatment decisions." *American Journal of Medicine* 92.2 (1992): 121-124.

Forsythe, D. E. "Blaming the user in medical informatics: the cultural nature of scientific practice." In *Knowledge and society: the anthropology of science and technology*, edited by D. J. Hess and L. L. Layne, 95-111. Hampton Hill: JAI Press, 1992.

Foucault, M. *The history of sexuality*. London: Tavistock, 1979.

Foucault, M. *Die Geburt der Klinik*. Frankfurt a. M.: Fischer, 1996.

Foucault, M. *Botschaften der Macht. Reader Diskurs und Medien*. Stuttgart: Deutsche Verlags-Anstalt, 1999.

Fox, R. C. "Training for uncertainty." In *The student-physician*, edited by R. K. Merton, G. Reader and P. L. Kendall, 207-241. Cambridge: Harvard University Press, 1957.

Fox, R. C. "The evolution of medical uncertainty." *Milbank Memorial Fund Quarterly* 58.1 (1980): 1-49.

Francioli, P. "Die Schweizerische HIV-Kohortenstudie/Swiss HIV Cohort Study (SHCS): Struktur und Funktionsweise." *Aids-Forschung Schweiz* 2 (1999): 42-44.

Fugelli, P. "Clinical practice: between Aristotle and Cochrane." *Schweizerische Medizinische Wochenschrift* 128.6 (1998): 184-188.

Fujimura, J. H. "Authorizing knowledge in science and anthropology." *American Anthropologist* 100.2 (1998): 347-360.

Fujimura, J. H., and D. W. Chou. "Dissent in science: styles of scientific practice and the dissent over the cause of AIDS." *Social Science and Medicine* 38.8 (1994): 1017-1036.

Gaines, A. D., and R. Hahn, eds. *Physicians of Western medicine: anthropological approaches to theory and practice*. Dordrecht: D. Reidel, 1985.

Generalsekretariat der Verbindung der Schweizer Ärztinnen und Ärzte FMH. "FMH Ärztestatistik 1998." *Schweizerische Ärztezeitung* 80.15 (1999): Sonderdruck.

Giddens, A. *The constitution of society: outline of the theory of structuration*. Cambridge: Polity Press, 1984.

Giddens, A. *Modernity and self-identity*. Cambridge: Polity Press, 1991.

Gilman, S. L. *Disease and representation: images of illness from madness to AIDS*. Ithaca: Cornell University Press, 1988.

Gold, R. S., J. Hinchy, and C. G. Batrouney. "The reasoning behind decisions not to take up antiretroviral therapy in Australians infected with HIV." *International Journal of STD and AIDS* 11.6 (2000): 361-370.

Goldstein, J. "Desperately seeking science: the creation of knowledge in family practice." *Hastings Center Report* 20.6 (1990): 26-32.

Good, B. J. *Medicine, rationality and experience: an anthropological perspective*. Cambridge: Cambridge University Press, 1994.

Good, B. J., and M.-J. DelVecchio Good. ""Learning medicine": the construction of medical knowledge at Harvard Medical School." In *Knowledge, power and practice: the anthropology of medicine and everyday life*, edited by S. Lindenbaum and M. Lock, 81-107. Berkeley: University of California Press, 1993.

Gordon, C. *Power/knowledge: selected interviews & other writings 1972-1977 by Michel Foucault*. New York: Pantheon Book, 1980.

Gordon, D. "Clinical science and clinical expertise: changing boundaries between art and science in medicine." In *Biomedicine examined*, edited by M. Lock and D. Gordon, 257-295. Dordrecht: Kluwer Academic Publishers, 1988.

Grahame-Smith, D. "Evidence based medicine: Socratic dissent." *British Medical Journal* 310.6987 (1995): 1126-1127.

Greene, S. "Science research and philanthropy. Government funding dominant." *Nature* 364.6439 (1993): 741-742.

Grimshaw, J. ""Life" for a non-progressor." *AIDS Care* 7.Supplement 1 (1994): S5-S9.

Grolle, J. "Sieg über die Seuche?" *Der Spiegel* 2 (1997): 118-124.

Grossman, Z., M. Polis, M. B. Feinberg, et al. "Ongoing HIV dissemination during HAART." *Nature Medicine* 5.10 (1999): 1099-1104.

Grun, L., and E. Murray. "Acceptability of shared care of asymptomatic HIV-positive patients." *Family Practice* 12.3 (1995): 299-302.

Gupta, A., and J. Ferguson. "Discipline and practice: "the field" as site, method, and location in anthropology." In *Anthropological locations: boundaries and grounds of a field science*, edited by A. Gupta and J. Ferguson, 1-46. Berkeley: University of California Press, 1997.

Hagendijk, R. "Structuration theory, constructivism, and scientific change." In *Theories of science in society*, edited by S. E. Cozzens and T. F. Gieryn, 43-66. Bloomington: Indiana University Press, 1990.

Hahn, R. A. *Sickness and healing: an anthropological perspective.* New Haven: Yale University Press, 1995.

Haines, A. "Guidance on guidelines. Writing them is easier than making them work." *British Medical Journal* 305.6857 (1992): 785-786.

Hall, J. A., D. L. Roter, and N. R. Katz. "Meta-analysis of correlates of provider behavior in medical encounters." *Medical Care* 26.7 (1988): 657-675.

Haraway, D. "The biopolitics of postmodern bodies: determinants of self in immune system discourse." *Differences* 1.1 (1989): 13-43.

Harley, A., J. D. Davids, J. M. Maskovsky, et al. Do people fail drugs, or do drugs fail people: the discourse of "adherence". 12th World AIDS Conference, Geneva (1998): 34212.

Harr, T., J. von Overbeck, C. Kopp, et al. "CD95 (fas)-expression on CD4- and CD8-lymphocytes of progressors and non-progressors to AIDS." *Journal of Clinical Microbiology and Infection* 3.Suppl. 2 (1997): P1051.

Hassin, J. "Living a responsible life: the impact of AIDS on the social identity of intravenous drug users." *Social Science and Medicine* 39.3 (1994): 391-400.

Hayes-Batistuta, D. E. "Modifying the treatment: patient compliance, patient control and medical care." *Social Science and Medicine* 10 (1976): 233-238.

Haynes, R. B. "Introduction." In *Compliance in health care*, edited by R. B. Haynes, D. W. Taylor and D. L. Sackett, 2. Baltimore: Johns Hopkins University, 1979.

Helman, C. G. *Culture, health and illness. An introduction for health professionals.* Oxford: Butterworth-Heinemann, 1994.

Herdt, G. "Introduction." In *The time of AIDS: social analysis, theory, and method*, edited by G. Herdt and S. Lindenbaum, 3-27. London: Sage Publications, 1992.

Herzlich, C. "Modern medicine and the quest for meaning: illness as a social signifier." In *Meaning of illness: anthropology, history, and sociology*, edited by M. Augé, C. Herzlich and K. Durnin, 151-173: Harwood Academic Publishers, 1995.

Hess, D. J. "Introduction: the new ethnography and the anthropology of science and technology." In *Knowledge and society: the anthropology of science and technology*, edited by D. J. Hess and L. L. Layne, 1-26. Hampton Hill: JAI Press, 1992.

Hirsch, E. "Aids: Neue ethische Dimensionen?" In *Neue Aids-Medikamente - neue ethische Probleme?*, edited by Aids Info Docu Schweiz, 19-25. Bern: Aids Info Docu Schweiz, 1997.

Hjortdahl, P., and E. Laerum. "Continuity of care in general practice: effects on patient satisfaction." *British Medical Journal* 304.6837 (1992): 1287-1290.

Ho, D. D. "Time to hit HIV, early and hard." *The New England Journal of Medicine* 333.7 (1995): 450-451.

Ho, D. D., A. U. Neumann, A. S. Perelson, et al. "Rapid turnover of plasma virions and CD4 lymphocytes in HIV-1 infection." *Nature* 373.6510 (1995): 123-126.

Hogg, R. S., A. E. Weber, K. J. P. Craib, et al. "One world, one hope: the costs of providing antiretroviral therapy to all nations." *AIDS* 12.16 (1998): 2203-2209.

Honkasalo, M.-L., and J. Lindquist. "An interview with Arthur Kleinman." *Ethnos* 62.3-4 (1997): 107-126.

Huby, G. "Interpreting silence, documenting experience: an anthropological approach to the study of health service users' experience with HIV/AIDS care in Lothian, Scotland." *Social Science and Medicine* 44.8 (1997): 1149-1160.

Huby, G., M. Porter, and J. Bury. "A matter of methods: perspectives on the role of the British general practitioner in the care of people with HIV/AIDS." *Aids Care* 10.Suppl. 1 (1998): S83-S88.

Hunt, L. M., and C. Mattingly. "Diverse rationalities and multiple realities in illness and healing." *Medical Anthropology Quarterly* 12.3 (1998): 267-272.

Hydén, L.-C. "Illness and narrative." *Sociology of Health and Illness* 19.1 (1997): 48-69.

Illich, I. "Pathogenese des Gesundheitswahns." *Le monde diplomatique*, April 1999, 3.

Jamous, H., and B. Peloille. "Changes in the French university-hospital system." In *Professions and professionalization*, edited by J. A. Jackson, 111-152. Cambridge: Cambridge University Press, 1970.

Johnson, H. J. "Dr. David Ho - The Lazarus equation." *Rolling Stone*, March 6 1997, 49-58, 84-89.

Jones, J. W. "Discourses of AIDS in West Germany, 1986-90." *Journal of the History of Sexuality* 2.3 (1992): 439-468.

Kaufert, P. "Menopause as process or event: the creation of definitions in biomedicine." In *Biomedicine examined*, edited by M. Lock and D. Gordon, 331-349. Dordrecht: Kluwer Academic Publishers, 1988.

Kaufman, S. R. "Toward a phenomenology of boundaries in medicine: chronic illness experience in the case of stroke." *Medical Anthropology Quarterly* 2.4 (1988): 338-354.

Kidd, M. "HIV management in general practice." *Australian Family Physician* 26.7 (1997): 779.

Kiefl, W. *Sozialwissenschaftliche Aids-Forschung. Anstösse für ein multimethodisches Paradigma.* Regensburg: S. Roderer, 1991.

King, M., R. Petchey, S. Singh, et al. "The role of the general practitioner in the community care of people with HIV infection and AIDS: A comparative study of high- and low-prevalence areas in England." *British Journal of General Practice* 48.430 (1998): 1233-1236.

Kirk, O., A. Mocroft, T. L. Katzenstein, et al. "Changes in use of antiretroviral therapy in regions of Europe over time." *AIDS* 12.15 (1998): 2031-2039.

Kirp, D. L., and R. Bayer, eds. *AIDS in the industrialized democracies: passions, politics, and policies.* New Brunswick: Rutgers, 1992.

Kitahata, M. M., T. D. Koepsell, R. A. Deyo, et al. "Physicians' experience with the Acquired Immunodeficiency Syndrome as a factor in patients' survival." *The New England Journal of Medicine* 334.11 (1996): 701-706.

Kleinman, A. *Patients and healers in the context of culture.* Berkeley: University of California Press, 1980.

Kleinman, A. *The illness narratives.* New York: Basic Books, 1988.

Kleinman, A. *Writing at the margin: discourse between anthropology and medicine.* Berkeley: University of California Press, 1995.

Koenig, B. A. "The technological imperative in medical practice: the social creation of a "routine" treatment." In *Biomedicine examined*, edited by M. Lock and D. Gordon, 465-495. Dordrecht: Kluwer Academic Publishers, 1988.

Köneke, S. *AIDS in der Presse. Der schreibende Umgang mit dem Ungewissen.* Freiburg i.B.: Universität Freiburg, 1991.

Kopp, C. "Neither here nor there: the anthropologist back from the clinic." *Tsantsa - Zeitschrift des Schweizerischen Ethnologischen Gesellschaft* .5 (2000): 128-132.

Kopp, C. "Know your risk." In *Tagungsbeiträge "Ordnung, Risiko und Gefährdung"*, edited by J. Rolshoven, A. Boscoboinik and C. Giordano, forthcoming. Freiburg: Freiburger Universitätsverlag, 2002.

Kopp, C., and S. Lang. "Neue Betreuungsmodelle für neue Lebensperspektiven." *Unipress*, Oktober 1999, 32-34.

Kopp, C., S. Lang, A. Iten, et al. From guidelines to clinical reality: doctors' and patients' views of health care and treatment in HIV. 12th World AIDS Conference, Geneva (1998a): 42293.

Kopp, C., S. Lang, A. Iten, et al. Betreuung und Therapiewahl bei HIV. Bern: Institut für Ethnologie, 1998b.

Kopp, C., S. Lang, and J. von Overbeck. "Soziodemographie und Lebensweise in einer schweizerischen Studie zur HIV-Nonprogression." *Schweizerische Medizinische Wochenschrift* 129.39 (1999): 1397-1404.

Laine, C., L. E. Markson, L. J. McKee, et al. "The relationship of clinic experience with advanced HIV and survival of women with AIDS." *AIDS* 12.4 (1998): 417-424.

Lambert, H., and H. Rose. "Disembodied knowledge? Making sense of medical science." In *Misunderstanding science? The public reconstruction of science and technology*, edited by A. Irwin and B. Wynne, 65-83. New York: Cambridge University Press, 1996.

Lang, S., C. Kopp, B. Federspiel, et al. The Swiss HIV Non Progressor Study - participant-centered study design as research strategy. XI International Conference on AIDS, Vancouver (1996): Mo. D. 1880.

Lang, S., C. Kopp, B. Federspiel, et al. Nutzung und Beurteilung von Betreuungsangeboten in einer Kohorte von asymptomatischen HIV long-term survivors. SGIM Jahresversammlung, Lausanne (1998): P95.

Latour, B., and S. Woolgar. *Laboratory life: the construction of scientific facts.* Princeton: Princeton University Press, 1986.

Le Pen, C. *Les habits neufs d'Hippocrate. Du médecin artisan au médecin ingénieur.* Paris: Calmann-Lévy, 1999.

Ledergerber, B., J. von Overbeck, M. Egger, et al. "The Swiss HIV Cohort Study: Rationale, organization and selected baseline characteristics." *Sozial- und Präventivmedizin* 39.6 (1994): 387-394.

Lee, B., and L. J. Montaner. "Chemokine immunobiology in HIV-1 pathogenesis." *Journal of Leukocyte Biology* 65.5 (1999): 552-565.

Levenstein, J., J. McCracken, I. McWhinney, et al. "The patient-centered clinical method. A model for the doctor-patient interaction in family practice." *Family Practice* 3.1 (1986): 24-30.

Lewis, C. E. "Management of patients with HIV/AIDS: who should care?" *JAMA* 278.14 (1997): 1133-1134.

Lock, M. "Introduction." In *Biomedicine examined*, edited by M. Lock and D. Gordon, 3-10. Dordrecht: Kluwer Academic Publishers, 1988.

Lock, M. "Cultivating the body: anthropology and epistemologies of bodily practice and knowledge." *Annual Review of Anthropology* 22 (1993a): 133-155.

Lock, M. *Encounters with aging: mythologies of menopause in Japan and North America.* Berkeley: University of California Press, 1993b.

Logan, R. L., and P. J. Scott. "Uncertainty in clinical practice: implications for quality and costs of health care." *The Lancet* 347.9001 (1996): 595-598.

Lüthi, T. "Von der Euphorie zum neuen Realismus." *Neue Zürcher Zeitung*, 8. Juli 1998, 68.

Maddox, J. "The prevalent distrust of science." *Nature* 378.6556 (1995): 435-437.

Madge, S., A. Mocroft, A. Olaitan, et al. "Do women with HIV infection consult with their GPs?" *British Journal of General Practice* 48.431 (1998): 1329-1330.

Malinverni, R., M. Müller, and N. E. Billo. "HIV Infektion: Umfrage bei praktizierenden Berner Ärzten." *Schweizerische Medizinische Wochenschrift* 122.26 (1992): 993-1004.

Mansfield, S., and S. Singh. "Who should fill the care gap in HIV disease?" *The Lancet* 342.8873 (1993): 726-728.

Marcus, G. E. "Ethnography in/of the world system: the emergence of multi-sited ethnography." *Annual Review of Anthropology* 24 (1995): 95-117.

Marcus, G. E., and M. M. J. Fischer. *Anthropology as cultural critique: an experimental moment in the human sciences.* Chicago: University of Chicago Press, 1986.

Martin, E. "Toward an anthropology of immunology: the body as nation state." *Medical Anthropology Quarterly* 4.4 (1990): 411-426.

Martin, E. "Body narratives, body boundaries." In *Cultural studies*, edited by L. Grossberg, C. Nelson and P. A. Treichler, 409-419. London: Routledge, 1992a.

Martin, E. "The end of the body?" *American Ethnologist* 19.1 (1992b): 120-138.

Martin, E. *Flexible bodies. The role of immunity in American culture from the days of Polio to the age of AIDS.* Boston: Beacon Press, 1994.

Martin, E. "The body at work: boundaries and collectivities in the late twentieth century." In *The social and political body*, edited by T. R. Schatzki and W. Natter, 145-157. New York: Guilford Press, 1996a.

Martin, E. "Citadels, rhizomes, and string figures." In *Technoscience and cyberculture*, edited by S. Aronowitz, 97-109. London: Routledge, 1996b.

Martin, E. "Anthropology and the cultural study of science: from citadels to string figures." In *Anthropological locations: boundaries and grounds of a field science*, edited by A. Gupta and J. Ferguson, 131-146. Berkeley: University of California Press, 1997.

Maskovsky, J. "Scheitern die Patienten oder die Medikamente?" *Aids Infothek* 5 (1998): 13-18.

Mattingly, C. "In search of the good: narrative reasoning in clinical practice." *Medical Anthropology Quarterly* 12.3 (1998): 273-297.

Mazumdar, P. M. H. *Species and specificity: an interpretation of the history of immunology*. Cambridge: Cambridge University Press, 1995.

McKee, M., and A. Clarke. "Guidelines, enthusiasm, uncertainty, and the limits to purchasing." *British Medical Journal* 310.6972 (1995): 101-104.

Meystre-Agustoni, G., F. Dubois-Arber, P. Cochand, et al. "Antiretroviral therapies from the patient's perspective." *AIDS Care* 12.6 (2000): 717-721.

Mishler, E. *The discourse of medicine: dialectics of medical interviews*. Norwood: Ablex, 1984.

Munzenberger, N., J. P. Cassuto, J. A. Gastaut, et al. "L'observance au cours des essais thérapeutiques dans l'infection VIH." *Presse Médicale* 26.8 (1997): 358-365.

Murray, S., and K. W. Payne. "The social classification of AIDS in American epidemiology." *Medical Anthropology* 10.2-3 (1989): 115-128.

Naylor, C. D. "Grey zones of clinical practice: some limits to Evidence-Based Medicine." *The Lancet* 345.8953 (1995): 840-842.

Naylor, C. D., E. Chen, and B. Strauss. "Measured enthusiasm: does the method of reporting trial results alter perceptions of therapeutic effectiveness?" *Annals of Internal Medicine* 117.11 (1992): 916-921.

Oppenheimer, G. M. "Causes, cases and cohorts: the role of epidemiology in the history of AIDS." In *AIDS: the making of a chronic disease*, edited by E. Fee and D. M. Fox, 49-83. Berkeley: University of California Press, 1992.

Orton, P. "Shared care." *The Lancet* 344.8934 (1994): 1413-1415.

Paauw, D., M. Weinrich, I. Curtis, et al. "Ability of primary care physicians to recognize physical findings associated with HIV infection." *JAMA* 274.17 (1995): 1380-1382.

Pantaleo, G., S. Menzo, M. Vaccarezza, et al. "Studies in subjects with long-term nonprogressive Human Immunodeficiency Virus infection." *New England Journal of Medicine* 332.4 (1995): 209-216.

Parson, T. *The social system*. New York: The Free Press, 1951.

Patton, C. *Inventing AIDS*. New York: Routledge, 1990.

Payer, L. *Medicine and culture: varieties of treatment in the United States, England, West Germany, and France*. New York: Henry Holt and Company, 1988.

Pécoul, B., P. Chirac, P. Trouiller, et al. "Access to essential drugs in poor countries - a lost battle?" *JAMA* 281.4 (1999): 361-367.

Perelson, A. S., P. Essunger, Y. Cao, et al. "Decay characteristics of HIV-1 infected compartments during combination therapy." *Nature* 387.6629 (1997): 188-191.

Perelson, A. S., P. Essunger, M. Markowitz, et al. How long should treatment be given if we had an antiretroviral agent that completely blocks HIV replication? 11th International Conference on AIDS, Vancouver (1996): Th. B. 930.

Pierce, D. R. "On outliving your friends." *AIDS Clinical Care* 2.1 (1990).

Pierret, J. "Un objet pour la sociologie de la maladie chronique: la situation de séropositivité au VIH?" *Sciences Sociales et Santé* 15.4 (1997): 97-120.

Pill, R., and N. C. H. Stott. "Concepts of illness causation and responsibility: some preliminary data from a sample of working class mothers." *Social Science and Medicine* 16.1 (1982): 43-52.

Pill, R., and N. C. H. Stott. "Development of a measure of potential health behaviour: a salience of lifestyle index." *Social Science and Medicine* 24.2 (1987): 125-134.

Pratt, M. L. "Fieldwork in common places." In *Writing culture: the poetics and politics of ethnography*, edited by J. Clifford and G. Marcus, 27-50. Berkeley: University of California Press, 1986.

Quam, M. D. "The sick role, stigma, and pollution: the case of AIDS." In *Culture and AIDS*, edited by D. A. Feldman, 29-44. New York: Praeger, 1990.

Rabinow, P. "Severing the ties: fragmentation and dignity in late modernity." In *Knowledge and society: the anthropology of science and technology*, edited by D. J. Hess and L. L. Layne, 169-187. Hampton Hill: JAI Press, 1992.

Radley, A. *Making sense of illness. The social psychology of health and disease*. London: Sage Publications, 1994.

Ramratnam, B., J. E. Mittler, L. Zhang, et al. "The decay of the latent reservoir of replication-competent HIV-1 is inversely correlated with the extent of residual viral replication during prolonged anti-retroviral therapy." *Nature Medicine* 6.1 (2000): 82-85.

Redijk, M., P. J. E. Bindels, J. Mohrs, et al. "Changing attitudes towards antiretroviral treatment of HIV infection: a prospective study in a sample of Dutch general practitioners." *AIDS Care* 11.2 (1999): 141-145.

Redijk, M., J. Mohrs, P. J. E. Bindels, et al. Initiation of antiretroviral treatment: decision-making in general practice. 12th World AIDS Conference, Geneva (1998): 60310.

Reeder, L. G. "The patient-client as consumer: some observations on the changing professional-client relationship." *Journal of Health and Social Behavior* 13.4 (1972): 406-412.

Ritschard, B. "Heute könnte es zum Durchbruch kommen." *Der Bund*, 2. Februar 2000, 13.

Rondeau, C. *De Sesam-Vitale à l'Internet, quels outils, quels Hippocrates à l'aube de l'XXI siècle*. Université d'Aix-Marseille: Faculté de Droit et de Sciences Publiques, 1999.

Rosenberg, W., and A. Donald. "Evidence based medicine: an approach to clinical problem-solving." *British Medical Journal* 310.6987 (1995): 1122-1126.

Rosenbrock, R., F. Dubois-Arber, M. Moers, et al. "The normalization of AIDS in Western European countries." *Social Science and Medicine* 50.11 (2000): 1607-1623.

Rouse, J. "What are cultural studies of scientific knowledge?" *Configurations* 1.1 (1992): 1-22.

Rutherford, G. "The Cochrane Collaboration and HIV/AIDS." *IAS Newsletter* 10 (1998): 14.

Sackett, D. L., and R. J. Cook. "Understanding clinical trials. What measures of efficacy should journal articles provide busy clinicians?" *British Medical Journal* 309.6957 (1994): 755-756.

Sackett, D. L., R. B. Haynes, G. H. Guyatt, et al. *Clinical epidemiology. A basic science for clinical medicine*. Boston: Little, Brown and Company, 1991.

Sackett, D. L., W. S. Richardson, W. Rosenberg, et al. *Evidence-Based Medicine*. New York: Churchill Livingstone, 1997.

Samuels, J. E. "Can IVDUs comply with conventional HIV care?" *AIDS Clinical Care* 2.4 (1990).

Samuels, J. E., J. Hendrix, M. Hilton, et al. "Zidovudine therapy in an inner city population." *Journal of Acquired Immune Deficiency Syndromes* 3.9 (1990): 877-883.

Sande, M. A., D. M. Gilbert, and R. C. Moellering. *The Sanford guide to HIV/AIDS therapy 1998*. Hyde Park: Antimicrobal Therapy, Inc., 1998.

Scheper-Hughes, N. "Embodied knowledge: thinking with the body in critical medical anthropology." In *Assessing cultural anthropology*, edited by R. Borofsky, 229-239. New York: McGraw Hill, 1994.

Scheper-Hughes, N., and M. Lock. "The mindful body: a prolegomenon to future work in medical anthropology." *Medical Anthropology Quarterly* 1.1 (1987): 6-41.

Schmittdiel, J., J. V. Selby, K. Grumbach, et al. "Choice of a personal physician and patient satisfaction in a Health Maintenance Organization." *JAMA* 278.19 (1997): 1596-1599.

Schrager, L. K., J. M. Young, M. G. Fowler, et al. "Long-term survivors of HIV-1 infection: definitions and research challenges." *AIDS* 8.supplement 1 (1994): S95-S108.

Schulz, T. *Kulturelle Konstruktion von AIDS: wissenschaftliche Erkenntnisproduktion und subjektive Deutung*. Frankfurt-Bockenheim: VAS, 1998.

Schwartz, R. K., S. B. Soumerai, and J. Avorn. "Physician motivations for nonscientific drug prescribing." *Social Science and Medicine* 28.6 (1989): 577-582.

Sennhauser, P. "Klares Ja zum neuen Arzttarif." *Der Bund*, 3. Februar 2000, 14.

Sheldon, J., E. Murray, A. Johnson, et al. "The involvement of general practitioners in the care of patients with Human Immunodeficiency Virus infection: current practice and future implications." *Family Practice* 10.4 (1993): 396-399.

Shilling, C. *The body and social theory.* London: Sage Publications, 1993.

Silverman, D., and M. Bloor. "Patient-centered medicine: some sociological observations on its constitution, penetration, and cultural assonance." In *Advances in medical sociology,* edited by G. L. Albrecht, 3-25. Greenwich: JAI Press, 1990.

Singer, M. *Critical medical anthropology.* Amityville: Baywood Publishing Company, 1995.

SKK/EKAF. "Neue Empfehlungen zur Behandlung der HIV-Infektion bei Erwachsenen." *BAG Bulletin* 20 (1997): 9-10.

SKK/EKAF. "Neue Empfehlungen zur Behandlung der HIV-Infektion bei Erwachsenen." *BAG Bulletin* 44 (1998).

Skultans, V. "Narrative illness and the body." *Anthropology and Medicine* 7.1 (2000): 5-12.

Smith, D., L. Goggin, H. Meldrum, et al. "Capturing the paradigm shift in HIV treatment: changing attitudes in the choice of combination antiretroviral drugs by high HIV caseload Australian GPs (1996-1997)." *AIDS Care* 12.1 (2000): 41-47.

Soloway, B. "A new era in HIV care." *American Family Physician* 56.1 (1997): 37, 40-42.

Speich, R. "Der diagnostische Prozess in der Inneren Medizin: Entscheidungsanalyse oder Intuition?" *Schweizerische Medizinische Wochenschrift* 127.31-32 (1997): 1263-1279.

Spiro, H. "What is empathy and can it be taught?" *Annals of Internal Medicine* 116.10 (1992): 843-846.

Stacey, M. "The naked truth." *American Photo* September/October (1999): 36-37.

Stimson, G. V. "Obeying doctor's orders: a view from the other side." *Social Science and Medicine* 8.2 (1974): 97-104.

Strathern, A. *Body thoughts.* Ann Arbor: University of Michigan Press, 1996.

Taussig, M. T. "Reification and the consciousness of the patient." *Social Science and Medicine* 14B.1 (1980): 3-13.

Thacker, S. B. "Meta-analysis. A quantitative approach to research integration." *JAMA* 259.11 (1988): 1685-1689.

Therrien, R., A. Gagnon, M. Mailhot, et al. Increasing patient adherence: experience with the "HIV medication guide". 12 World AIDS Conference, Geneva (1998): 32369.

Treichler, P. A. "AIDS, HIV, and the cultural construction of reality." In *The time of AIDS: social analysis, theory, and method,* edited by G. Herdt and S. Lindenbaum, 65-98. London: Sage Publications, 1992.

Trostle, J. A. "Medical compliance as an ideology." *Social Science and Medicine* 27.12 (1988): 1299-1308.

Trutmann, M., and R. Steiner. "Können Sie noch ruhig schlafen, Herr Präsident?" *Schweizerische Ärztezeitung* 46 (1999).

Turner, B. S. *Medical power and social knowledge.* London: Sage Publications, 1995.

Turner, V. *The ritual process.* Ithaca: Cornell University Press, 1969.

van der Geest, S., S. Reynolds White, and A. Hardon. "The anthropology of pharmaceuticals: a biographical approach." *Annual Review of Anthropology* 25 (1996): 153-178.

Varmus, H. E. "Naming the AIDS virus." In *The meaning of AIDS: implications for medical science, clinical practice, and public health policy,* edited by E. T. Juengst and B. A. Koenig, 3-11. New York: Praeger Publishers, 1989.

Veldhuis, M. "Defensive behaviour of Dutch family physicians. Widening the concept." *Family Medicine* 26.1 (1994): 27-29.

Veldhuis, M., L. Wigersma, and I. Okkes. "Deliberate departures from good general practice: a study of motives among Dutch general practitioners." *British Journal of General Practice* 48.437 (1998): 1833-1836.

Venrath, B. *AIDS. Die soziale Definition einer Krankheit.* Oldenburg: BIS, 1994.

Verbindung der Schweizer Ärzte. "Mitglieder-Statistik 1988 der Verbindung der Schweizer Ärzte." *Schweizerische Ärztezeitung* 70.23 (1988): Separatdruck.

Viciana, P., M. Dolores Prados, G. Gomez Vera, et al. "Buffalo hump" associated with protease inhibitors and use of corticoids ointment. 12th World AIDS Conference, Geneva (1998): 12403.

Walker, B., and I. Waddington. "AIDS and the doctor-patient relationship." *Social Studies Review* 6.4 (1991): 128-130.

Wallston, K. A. "Development of the Multidimensional Health Locus of Control (MHLC) scales." *Health Education Monographs* 6.2 (1978): 160-170.

Webb, S., and M. Lloyd. "Prescribing and referral in general practice: a study of patients' expectations and doctors' actions." *British Journal of General Practice* 44.381 (1994): 165-169.

Weber, M. *Die protestantische Ethik und der "Geist" des Kapitalismus. Textausgabe auf Grundlage der ersten Fassung von 1904/05.* Bodenheim: Athenäum, 1993.

Whittaker, A. M. "Living with HIV: resistance by positive people." *Medical Anthropology Quarterly* 6.4 (1992): 385-390.

Wieland, W. "The concept of the art of medicine." In *Science, technology, and the art of medicine,* edited by C. Delkeskamp-Hayes and M. A. Gardell Cutter, 165-181. Dordrecht: Kluwer Academic Publishers, 1993.

Wigersma, L., S. Singh, and F. M. L. G. van den Boom. "Meeting the needs of those infected and affected by HIV/AIDS." *Aids Care* 10.Suppl. 1 (1998): S5-S8.

Williams, G. "The genesis of chronic illness: narrative re-construction." *Sociology of Health and Illness* 6.2 (1984): 175-200.

Wilson, D., P. Cawthorne, N. Ford, et al. "Global trade and access to medicines: AIDS treatments in Thailand." *The Lancet* 354.9193 (1999): 1893-1895.

Wilson Ross, J. "Ethics and the language of AIDS." In *The meaning of AIDS: implications for medical science, clinical practice, and public health policy,* edited by E. T. Juengst and B. A. Koenig, 30-40. New York: Praeger Publishers, 1989.

Winefield, H. R., T. G. Murrell, and J. Clifford. "Process and outcomes in general practice: problems in defining high quality care." *Social Science and Medicine* 41.7 (1995): 969-975.

Woolf, S. T. "Practice guidelines, a new reality in medicine: I. Recent developments." *Archives of Internal Medicine* 150.9 (1990): 1811-1818.

Woolf, S. T. "Practice guidelines, a new reality in medicine: II. Methods of developing guidelines." *Archives of Internal Medicine* 152.5 (1992): 946-952.

Woolf, S. T. "Practice guidelines, a new reality in medicine: III. Impact on patient care." *Archives of Internal Medicine* 153.23 (1993): 2646-2655.

Wright, A. L., and W. J. Morgan. "On the creation of "problem" patients." *Social Science and Medicine* 30.9 (1990): 951-959.

Young, B., and D. R. Kuritzkes. "Viral kinetics: implications for treatment." *AIDS* 13.suppl. 1 (1999): S11-S17.

Zola, I. K. "Pathways to the doctor - from person to patient." *Social Science and Medicine* 7.9 (1973): 677-689.

Zuger, A., and V. L. Sharp. "'HIV specialists': the time has come." *JAMA* 278.14 (1997): 1131-1132.

# INDEX

# International Library of Ethics, Law, and the New Medicine

KLUWER ACADEMIC PUBLISHERS – DORDRECHT / BOSTON / LONDON